T0279643

BEING ILL

BEING ILL

On Sickness, Care and Abandonment

Neil Vickers and Derek Bolton

REAKTION BOOKS

In memory of Aubrey Sheiham

Published by

REAKTION BOOKS LTD
Unit 32, Waterside
44–48 Wharf Road
London N1 7UX, UK

www.reaktionbooks.co.uk

First published 2024
Copyright © Neil Vickers and Derek Bolton 2024

Printed and bound in Great Britain
by Bell & Bain, Glasgow

A catalogue record for this book is available from the British Library

ISBN 978 1 78914 911 1

CONTENTS

Introduction
7

1 Emergent Illness
34

2 Care
72

3 The Pariah Syndrome
121

4 Biopsychosocial Beings
162

Conclusion
200

REFERENCES *219*
BIBLIOGRAPHY *243*
ACKNOWLEDGEMENTS *250*
INDEX *251*

Introduction

Amajor diagnosis changes how others see us, in ways that are difficult to control. Few if any relationships remain the same. Relations with intimate others often become closer as we become more dependent on them; more distant contacts become more strained; and, if the illness is visible, even relations with complete strangers may become fraught. If you are diagnosed with a major disease, you are likely to be dropped by at least some of your friends and acquaintances. If you're lucky, you will find that while people in the middle distance and further out move away, intimate others draw nearer. As the poet Anne Boyer remarked, 'people leave, friends drop off, lovers abscond with all possibility of you ever again being fond of them, colleagues avoid you, your rivals are now unimpressed, your Twitter followers unfollow.'[1]

There can be good reasons for the reconfiguring of relationships. A sick person might need to withdraw for a time from social contacts, and a healthy acquaintance might wish to give a sick person the privacy to get on with their life as best they can without interference. But, in the rich parts of the West at least, such decisions often become a slippery slope leading to the isolation of the ill. This book is about why and how that happens, and the collective dimensions of illness in societies committed to individualism.

No one has evoked this phenomenon more powerfully than the anthropologist S. Lochlann Jain, themselves the author of a fine memoir of cancer:

When my cousin Elise was undergoing chemotherapy treatment while in her early thirties, I couldn't even mention cancer, couldn't (wouldn't, didn't) say I was sorry or ask her how she was doing – even though it was so obviously what was going on. I was thirty-five, for God's sake, a grown-up, yet cancer was so unthinkable that I couldn't even acknowledge her disease. Whatever rationalizing spin I try to give it, I sucked in all the ways I had to deal with later when others made similar dumbish comments.[2]

This awkwardness around the sick often extends to their close others. The family members of people with major illnesses report that acquaintances and friends either avoid them completely, thereby imposing what sociologists call 'secondary stigma', or strike up conversations in which they do not mention the sick person. It is as if they had never existed. This latter phenomenon sometimes goes by the name of 'premature widow syndrome' but it is not confined to spouses. The children of sick people experience it too. They become a troublesome reminder of good intentions unfulfilled; or, as the poet Rachel Hadas puts it, they become 'the disturbance in the room'.[3]

In highlighting the relational and transpersonal dimensions of illness, we do not wish to minimize the importance of the illness for the individual. The toll illness can take on our sense of ourselves is often devastating. But the relational effects still warrant study because they are routinely denied. Most people are aware of the effects of major psychiatric disorders on relationships. But we are much slower to acknowledge the stigma of physical illness. There is little training for health professionals to deal with this phenomenon and there are few if any supports for family members and others who live with and support the ill.

First-person memoirs of illness and caring have a great deal to say about it. 'How does it feel', asks Rachel Hadas, whose husband began to develop frontotemporal dementia in his fifties, 'when people you thought were your friends turn away from illness?'[4] 'I do not want to imply or say that I have been deserted by all my friends and colleagues,' writes Albert Robillard, a sociologist afflicted with amyotrophic lateral sclerosis (ALS), known in the UK as motor neurone disease. 'In fact, a few friendships have become stronger during my illness. These few have offered and have delivered every kind of assistance to me and my wife, Divina.' Robillard is eloquent on the stigma arising from his illness: 'I see averted faces and the manifestation of overriding interactional involvements.'[5] Arthur W. Frank, the theorist of illness and storytelling, recalls that even before his cancer was diagnosed, when he was still only at the stage of medical investigation, some friends withdrew because they did not want to hear about even the possibility that he was seriously ill. So disturbed was Susan Sontag by the reactions of others to her breast cancer that she began to research the history of cultural meanings of that disease, and the result was her classic book *Illness as Metaphor* (1977). Back then, many cancer patients concealed their cancer from others because it was 'felt to be obscene – in the original sense of that word: ill-omened, abominable, repugnant to the senses.'[6]

One of the most striking literary accounts of this phenomenon is by Seamus Heaney in a poem, 'Miracle', written in 2005, shortly after his first stroke. The miracle of its title is the work not of the ill person, but of intimate others, 'the ones who have known him all along'. The fact that they are there at all is the miracle. The poem bears witness to the value of the very thing so many ill people are deprived of: continued familiarity.

We know, of course, that some people really do rise wonderfully to the challenge of illness in a relative, friend or colleague. People can and do behave kindly and graciously to the ill. But they are rarer than most people think. Neither would we wish to downplay the tremendous potential of collective social action. Indeed, one of the major themes of this book will be its importance. Organizations like the London Lighthouse and the Terrence Higgins Trust did an enormous amount of good by creating voluntary caring arrangements whereby a trained volunteer, known informally as a buddy, would agree to look after a person with AIDS by visiting them regularly, doing shopping for them and perhaps some housework, but mostly listening to them and witnessing what they were going through.[7]

Despite these inspirational exceptions, we nevertheless think that people in the affluent world do not make enough room for sickness or dying as part of life. It is not that we bear the sick and the dying ill will. That is very rarely the case. But, as the sociologist and disability activist Irving Zola put it, the sick must reckon with 'the sense of infirmity we evoke in others and their consequent incapacity to deal with us'.[8] This seems to account for a phenomenon Arthur Frank described well:

> Too many ill people are deprived of the experience of conversation . . . Ill persons have a great deal to say for themselves, but rarely do I hear them talk about their hopes and fears, about what it is like to be in pain, about what sense they make of suffering and the prospect of death. Because such talk embarrasses us, we do not have practice with it. Lacking practice, we find such talk difficult.[9]

Some patients have even written about the necessity of making a permanent break with the world of healthy strangers.

In some respects our culture seems more open to illness now than ever before. Newspaper columns by John Diamond, Ruth Picardie and Barbara Ehrenreich, for example, have taken much of the taboo out of the idea of illness. Bestsellers have been written about it, some of which have been turned into mass-market Hollywood films: Susanna Kaysen's book *Girl, Interrupted* (1993) was turned into a movie starring Winona Ryder, Angelina Jolie and Vanessa Redgrave in 1999; John Bayley's *Iris: A Memoir of Iris Murdoch* (1998) was adapted and released as a film in 2001, as was Jean-Dominique Bauby's *The Diving Bell and the Butterfly* (1997) in 2007. Some illness blogs, such as Kate Gross's 'The Nuisance: News from Kate's attic on life, and cancer. In that order', have attracted huge followings. Illness has almost become a branch of the entertainment industry. But there is a world of difference between being willing to read a book or watch a movie about the ills of strangers and staying in touch with a friend or acquaintance who has been struck down by a major illness. Robert McCrum has captured this paradox brilliantly:

> Oddly enough, the more everything is reported, analysed, expounded, categorised and explored in newspaper column after column, and the more people feel able to express whatever they think about virtually anything under the sun, the more deafening is the silence that hangs over illness and ill-health.[10]

The problem we are describing is especially acute in societies the anthropologist Joseph Henrich calls WEIRD: Western, educated, individualistic, rich and democratic.[11] This comprises the industrialized societies of North America, northwestern Europe and Oceania. It excludes eastern and southern Europe as well as all of Asia and Africa. Most people on the planet are, therefore, not WEIRD.

The acronym has been subjected to powerful critique and in using it we do not wish to endorse everything Henrich says about it.[12] But we do think the way WEIRD societies think about and handle illness is distinctive in certain respects. Such cultures are largely secular and encourage the individual to function as an atomized consumer in relation to his or her health; despite a rhetoric of community, they tend to drive the ill to the margins of society; and they have no idea how to integrate death into life meaningfully. They are largely committed to the idea of the sovereign individual and are bad at thinking about situations in which the self is not substantially in control of its own actions. Yet even a cursory survey of first-person accounts of major illness reveals that healthy people often behave in ways they would consider 'out of character' when confronted with a sick or potentially sick person. Many WEIRD societies contain pockets of non-WEIRDness. Religion is still a potent binding force in many working-class Irish communities, for example, and the response to illness accordingly follows a different pattern. Minority ethnic and religious communities throughout these societies also tend to handle illness differently.

Some readers may be wondering at this point if the problem we're describing might be peculiar to a very specific demographic, namely a subgroup of highly skilled writers of commercially published memoirs. It has to be acknowledged that the estrangement of the healthy from the ill has an odd academic status. Landmark articles have been written about it. Perhaps the most famous of these is by a neurologist whose case we discuss in Chapter Three, David Rabin.[13] When Rabin was struck down by motor neurone disease, he found that he and his family were treated like pariahs by their colleagues and friends. He called the problem 'the pariah syndrome'. With his wife Pauline, a psychiatrist, he published a book relating other sick physicians' experiences of the pariah syndrome. The relatives of the sick have also written especially movingly about it.[14]

Yet the estrangement of the healthy from the ill does not form a distinct or a discrete area of academic research. There are several literatures dealing with aspects of the problem, but none offers a systematic or syncretic overview.

Here is a very brief overview of the academic status of the subject. Studies of isolation in illness often treat it as if it were solely the result of the limitations imposed by the health condition.[15] The role of the healthy and the able-bodied in bringing about isolation usually isn't mentioned.

There is a gigantic sociological literature on stigma, including health stigma. The foundational text remains Erving Goffman's *Stigma: Notes on the Management of Spoiled Identity* (1963).[16] It is grist to our mill that around two-thirds of Goffman's examples of stigma concern sick or disabled individuals. Until HIV was brought under control through combination therapies, there was a substantial literature on the stigma of AIDS, but as HIV infection has become a completely disguisable (and treatable) condition in WEIRD societies, this is no longer the case. Today, the literature on health stigma is dominated by studies of the stigma of mental illness.

There is also a fascinating epidemiological literature on the *consequences* of stigma. In recent years, this literature has become increasingly preoccupied by the ways in which social discrimination of various kinds negatively impacts health.[17] And there is a related but distinct literature detailing the ways in which loneliness and social isolation (which are not always caused by stigma) increase the risk of disease and death.[18]

There is a substantial condition-based literature on the stigma attaching to chronic physical illnesses of various kinds (endometriosis, fibromyalgia, lupus, asthma, epilepsy and diabetes), which focuses on how people with these conditions mask them from the healthy.[19] Today, this literature is dominated by social psychologists, though it has deep roots in the work of sociologists, notably Goffman.

One of the most interesting treatments of the problem is by writers interested in death.[20] This body of research emphasizes the irrationality surrounding the fear of the dying, especially in the secular West. The sick as dying or potentially dying people unwittingly provoke this irrational response.

Two areas of scholarship tackle it directly. The first is evolutionary psychology. Evolutionary psychologists argue that the isolation of the ill is the result of an adaptation that occurred during the Pleistocene era when there would have been strong survival incentives 'to avoid poor social exchange partners, join cooperative groups (for purposes of between-group competition and exploitation), and avoid contact with those who are differentially likely to carry communicable pathogens'.[21] The second is disability studies. The contrast between the literatures on disability and sickness could hardly be greater in respect of the question of isolation. Disability theorists have demonstrated very powerfully how difficult it can be for the able-bodied to give up normative assumptions about the body, assumptions that disabled people seldom live up to. The sick have not managed to fight back to the same extent. This matters because modern medicine's greatest achievement is, arguably, to have converted so many acute conditions into chronic ones. As the feminist philosopher Sarah Wendell observed, nowadays chronic diseases are effectively disabilities.[22] They are aetiologically complex. They are managed biomedically but usually there is no cure. As with disabilities, aetiological risks accumulate across the life span. And personal coping is crucial.

We propose to examine the problem by focusing mostly on the attitudes of the healthy in WEIRD societies towards major illness. In highly individualistic societies, there are reasons to be chary of becoming the sick person's main support. A sick person in all their vulnerability calls out to us as one human being to another. It is a piercing call, made more so by the fact that it is often impossible to know in advance what it may entail. Who would want to be the sick person's carer of last or only resort? This gives rise to a version of the problem Bibb Latané and John M. Darley explored in their celebrated book *The Unresponsive Bystander: Why Doesn't He Help?* (1970).[23] If more people came forward, bystanding wouldn't be so much of a problem. The issue is compounded by the fact that unresponsive bystanders are unresponsive not only to the person in need but to others who go to his or her aid.

'Health is a mode of omnipotence,' according to the physician-writer Eric Cassell, and we agree with him.[24] Of course, it's not *just* a mode of omnipotence, but it is also that. 'Health is a state of insouciance,' says the physician-philosopher Georges Canguilhem, making the same point in a less psychodynamic idiom.[25] What we take both these writers to mean is that the feeling of health is a highly defended state – defended, that is, against even the *knowledge* of illness.

The circumstances behind the writing of Elisabeth Kübler-Ross's *On Death and Dying: What the Dying Have to Teach Doctors, Nurses, Clergy, and Their Own Families* (1969) shed some light on this defendedness. Kübler-Ross was a psychoanalytically trained psychiatrist working at Billings Hospital, one of the main teaching hospitals associated with Chicago University. In 1965 she was approached by four theology students for help with a project on a 'crisis in human life'. The students had selected dying as their crisis but they weren't sure how to go about researching it. They knew they wanted to carry out an empirical study of some kind. Kübler-Ross suggested they interview dying patients at Billings.

> I set out to ask physicians of different services and wards for permission to interview a terminally ill patient of theirs. The reactions were varied, from stunned looks of disbelief to rather abrupt changes of topic of conversation; the end result being that I did not get one single chance even to get near such a patient. Some doctors 'protected' their patients by saying that they were too sick, too tired, or weak, or not the talking kind; others bluntly refused to take part in such a project.[26]

A few doctors eventually broke ranks and identified dying patients for her. Between 1965 and 1969, she and her team interviewed more than four hundred terminally ill patients. The vast majority had worked out that they were dying, but around half had never even been told they had a serious illness. These interviews formed the basis for *On Death and Dying*. Kübler-Ross is generally regarded as one of the first workers to try to get close to the experience of the ill. She came to the view that the denial of the patient's experience was rooted in the reluctance of the clinical staff to face it squarely, and, behind that, the denial in the society they served. Dying was, she said, a subject of generalized 'social repression'.[27] Facing the patient's death involves exposing oneself to his or her envy. It also involves facing one's own death, which entails relinquishing omnipotence and insouciance.

But there is also surely a bodily dimension at work too. Edmund Husserl, the founder of modern phenomenology, observed that our capacity to share experiences with others turns on a process by which we simulate their experiences in our own bodies. Merleau-Ponty suggested that this results in a situation where we believe that we perform the action we see others carry out. This was his famous theory of the 'shared body schema'.[28] It is almost as if he had anticipated the theory of mirror neurons. We might note in passing that the psychoanalytic theories of projection and introjection implicitly rely on a theory like the theory of the shared body schema, for these actions assume that psychobiological states can be passed from one body to another. The shared body schema, as Merleau-Ponty describes it, is a highly dynamic entity: as our perception of the other person changes moment by moment, different aspects of the shared body schema will move in and out of salience. We use others' bodily experiences as templates for our own, not only in a general way, but in the here and now, moment by moment. If I see someone who is paralysed, then in some sense I'm paralysed, and that constitutes a heavy blow to my omnipotence. But if there are other people in the vicinity to share the burden with me, I may hold my nerve better. The dying pose a particularly delicate challenge in this regard.

The anti-psychiatrist Thomas Szasz once remarked that 'in all close human relationships which are characterized by a high degree of mutual interdependence, the suffering and unhappiness of one member assumes a signal function for his partner.' He went on:

> This means that his suffering will signify not only that he is hurt or sick (which may or may not be the case) but also that his partner is *bad*, for he has failed to gratify his needs! Thus arises the more general idea that in all sorts of human relations one's partner's unhappiness or discomfort signifies *the badness of the self*.[29]

Extrapolating from Szasz's claim, we may wonder if the fear of being designated a bad carer has a pre-emptively discouraging effect on many people of good will. Perhaps at an unconscious level they think they are being asked to cure the sick other. This is especially the case in a culture that deals with illness in biomedical terms alone. If we try and fail to cure him or her, we expose ourselves to terrible guilt and shame. Our culture is beholden to the idea that biomedical support is what the sick need more than anything else. But the sick also need authentic contact. Authentic contact doesn't have to dwell exclusively on a poor prognosis. Some minimal acknowledgement is often enough. Yet what is striking in so many accounts of major illness is the frequency with which the healthy refuse even minimal acknowledgement.

A healthy person offers other healthy people a relatively stable set of assumptions that make interaction with them seem safe and rewarding. But life-changing illness changes perceptions of sick people in ways that can be hard to grasp all at once. It is all but inevitable that our shared intercorporeal and interaffective world will be shaken to its foundations. In his wonderful book *The Wounded Storyteller* (1995) Arthur Frank proposed storytelling as a stabilizing force – a position he has developed further in subsequent publications. In Frank's view, postmodern societies have alienated us from sick bodies. The sick 'need to become storytellers in order to recover the voices that illness and its treatment often take away'.[30] Frank is clear that the healthy and the able-bodied are often not ready to hear stories of sickness, and in his later work it can sometimes seem as if the most receptive audience for these stories are other sick people. The act of telling is one of which we warmly approve, but we don't think the absence of stories or even information is the main stumbling block preventing the sick and the healthy from remaining in contact. It has more to do with the sense of infirmity that illness evokes in both parties. It is a multistranded problem of *interaction* affecting both the healthy and the ill.

A biopsychosocial approach

This book is intended as a contribution to the medical or health humanities and, at the same time, an example of a direction in which we think the discipline can be profitably extended. We think the reach of the medical humanities can be extended significantly by the health sciences of the last forty years or so. These include the finding that the so-called social determinants of health – the conditions in which people are born, grow, live, work and age – account for the lion's share of inequalities in health outcomes; the discovery that social disadvantage becomes embedded in the body physiologically over and above any effects caused by individual lifestyle and behavioural factors; the increasing sophistication of systems biology; the development of modern neuroscience; and the development of epigenetics. If the medical humanities are to blossom, they need to engage not only with a wide range of critical theories (the 'secure base' of humanities and social science scholars everywhere) but with scientific discoveries like these. Very little work in the medical humanities today engages with the fact that humans are a sexually reproducing mammalian species endowed with specific motivational systems that, on average and over time, shape their behaviour in somewhat predictable ways and, no less significantly, affect their health. The social determinants of health have had almost no impact and neither has the long-term impact of childhood adversity. To take account of such matters is assumed – wrongly, in our view – to be deterministic and/or biologistic. Indeed, in some quarters, there is a shallow hostility to scientific and medical endeavour per se on the assumption that eugenics or something like it is just a heartbeat away.

An earlier generation of medical humanities scholars engaged with research in the health sciences to a much greater extent than is the case today through the biopsychosocial model of health and disease. People joining the medical humanities from the humanities or social sciences disciplines today often don't know what the biopsychosocial model is, or else they think it's a theory of medical practice. It has to be conceded that George Engel, the model's originator, applied the name very widely and did think that clinicians could learn to practice 'biopsychosocially'. But his first paper describing the model, which he published in 1977, makes clear that it is also – we would say first and foremost – a theory of health and disease causation. Biomedicine views illness solely in terms of biological insults and defects. The biopsychosocial model was an attempt to theorize the role of psychosocial factors in causing illness. While we have criticisms of Engel's model, and will be presenting in Chapter Four of this book a radically updated version that is in certain key respects different from his, we still think he got a lot right.

A biopsychosocial approach to any problem necessarily takes as its starting point humans' status as open biological systems in social environments. Self-evidently, the medical humanities have no monopoly on biopsychosocial thinking. Versions of biopsychosociality will also be familiar to readers acquainted with biologically oriented anthropology and sociology. We think the biopsychosocial model – appropriately updated to take account of the developments mentioned above – offers a remarkable source of transdisciplinary undergirding for the medical humanities, one that it will enable with a stake in the field to take part in a dialogue of equals.

WE PROPOSE IN this book to explore the problem of abandonment of the sick by the healthy by looking at our biopsychosocial nature. This involves two commitments. First, it requires us to pay special attention to the biological, psychological and social effects of ordinary human interactions. We call this our account of shared life, in effect an account of what human relatedness is like under conditions of health, and go on to explore some of the ways in which illness interferes with that norm. Second, it requires us to consider the longer-term effects on health of drawing nearer to and pulling away from other human beings. Our health is massively dependent on our being included in communal living. Studies in epidemiology, epigenetics and social neuroscience completed since the 1980s tell us that social adversity is bad for our health and can become embedded in the body physiologically, leading to greater risk of illness and death. This book attempts to place the response to illness in the rich world in the context of this work.

We draw on a wide panorama of academic disciplines in this book, but we owe a special debt to one discipline in particular: infant research, a supremely biopsychosocial specialty. Infant research is a field that sheds immense light on the question of what it is like to *be with* another person. Some readers may object that the 'being with' that caregiver–infant dyads do is worlds away from what goes on when two adults talk together, but we want to suggest that the microfoundations on which both types of communication arise are remarkably similar and that the parallels are especially illuminating when considering how the healthy interact with the ill.

One of the things infant research shows so magnificently is how deep emotional bonds emerge from interactions based on some form of reciprocity. The infant imitates the carer or engages in to-and-fro play with them and discovers a rich world of intersubjectivity that can be enlarged through other, often more sophisticated forms of reciprocity. This is the key to the unfolding of the young child's capacities.

Over time, two modes of intersubjectivity emerge. We evolve a transactionally based mode, founded on a highly delimited form of engagement with another person, alongside intersubjectivity of a more embedded kind, which we usually find among people who share large-scale life-projects with one another (marriage, child-rearing, the promotion of a particular religious or political vision of life and so on). Reciprocity is central in both.

These two different modes of intersubjectivity have been recognized in many recent disciplines. It is central to infant research, most of the major programmes in social neuroscience and 4E cognition, a new cross-disciplinary field that attempts to capture the dynamic interactions between the brain, body and both the physical and social environments. These more recent developments are all well anchored in Darwinian thought.

It is important to state from the outset that both modes are important. We have a need for close others from whom we can draw strength and to whom we can give support. And we also have a need to be acknowledged as creditable figures more generally, worthy of everything the groups to which we belong can offer us (which is one of the reasons why social exclusion is often so catastrophic in its effects). The kinds of creative interaction we can enjoy in each of these domains are sometimes very different from one another. They are inevitably shaped by culture and it therefore follows that the way the distinction between them is managed is also shaped by culture (though the separation of the two domains is probably rooted in our evolutionary history).

To home in on the peculiarities of these two areas – the distant and the intimate spheres of everyday life – we will borrow concepts from two thinkers who are seldom paired together: the American sociologist Erving Goffman (1922–1982) and the British paediatrician and psychoanalyst Donald Winnicott (1896–1971). Goffman was interested in how human beings interact in one another's presence. He called this face-to-face domain of group life 'the interaction order'. Winnicott was a student of how babies and children interact with their carers and the environment in which they receive care. He developed a highly original theory of what infants need in order to thrive, to which he gave the name 'holding'.[31] In Chapter One we will propose an extension of this theory and argue that 'holding' is something adults need too. Holding implies a supportive attitude, but the theory was elaborated to account for the consequences of an absence of support. As befits a paediatrician and a psychoanalyst, Winnicott was especially interested in the developmental and counter-developmental aspects of family life. He is a thinker most at home in the intimate sphere. It is striking how little Goffman has to say about intimate relationships.[32]

Broadly speaking, when we use Goffman, we shall be concerned with what might be termed 'the outside world': officialdom in all its forms (employers, schools, the healthcare system, social services, the police, the courts and so on) as well as relationships of a less stressful sort such as those we acquire through hobbies or interests. And when we use Winnicott, we shall be concerned with intimate others. Obviously, the matter is not completely clear-cut, for the two are overlapping, especially when we think of friends who can choose how much responsibility they wish to take for us. In such cases it behoves us to keep both conceptual frameworks in mind.

Goffman, inclined to the tragic, was viscerally alive to the inter-action order's destructive potential. He was also a more transactional thinker than Winnicott, often describing relationships in terms that seem to anticipate game theory. (He once remarked that 'gambling is a prototype of action.'[33]) Winnicott, by temperament an optimist, was concerned with the transformative potential of the holding environment and stresses the ways in which holding endows children with creative resources that go beyond the details of any single interaction. He emphasized in particular how holding makes possible the child's sense of spontaneity. Although both men acknowledged a psychobiological dimension in human interactions, Winnicott offered a more detailed and counterintuitive picture of how it works, and we will explore this at some length in Chapters One and Two.

The two perspectives are mostly complementary and both are necessary. Goffman teaches us to keep in mind the profoundly motivating character of the interaction order. Having a place in at least one interaction order gives us a default reason to go on living. He also lays useful stress on the fragility of the interaction order and on the need for the agreements that underlie it to be renewed constantly. Winnicott, on the other hand, as the theorist of quantum leaps in child development, stresses the powerful effect of love and deep interpersonal knowing on the holding environment to a degree that has no parallel in Goffman's work.

The interaction order and the holding environment form a continuum. Most interaction orders offer a minimum of holding and some offer considerably more. They both use signs of responsive recognition to initiate and maintain relationships of reciprocity. They both have marked physiological effects. Each involves – at least some of the time – what cognitive psychologists call 'high-engagement interactions'. High-engagement interactions require us, in Colwyn Trevarthen's words, to inhabit 'one mind-time and one body-related space' with another person.[34] We find ourselves in a kind of 'dance' of movements and sounds and affects with the other person or persons. A precondition for high-engagement interactions is that we have to suppress the physiologically costly responses of the sympathetic nervous system (the so-called fight–flight response). High engagement usually results in neurobiological coregulation with at least one other person. Our heart rates and breathing rates converge, and so do our cortisol levels. When this process works well, it enables us to draw physiological as well as psychological and emotional sustenance from another person or persons.

We said earlier that the holding environment and the interaction order are both important, and they are, but the holding environment is more fundamental. Infant research shows that babies cannot thrive without an experience of others 'locking on' to their minds. Without it, they develop autism-like symptoms. They have to undergo certain organizing experiences in the social world or else their living energies dissipate and, in the terms of Isabelle Stengers and Ilya Prigogine, they lose complexity and coherence as organisms. Their physical as well as their psychological development can be fatally compromised as a result; this is one of the findings of the studies of Romanian children who had been abandoned in orphanages during the Ceaușescu regime. All-cause mortality for Romanian orphans (that is to say death due to any cause) was much higher than that recorded for the rest of the Romanian population.

The Stengers–Prigogine vision potentially extends far beyond the nurturing of infants, for adults are also heavily reliant on organizing social experiences. This may explain, for instance, why loneliness is so bad for our health and why bereavement can affect us so deleteriously. People who are bereaved often report the sense of living in frozen time in the absence of the significant other. It is as if the mere presence of the other had provided a kind of scaffolding for their health that they hadn't noticed was there. When it is withdrawn, their health collapses.[35] That's a simple example. We might also think of the deleterious impact of unemployment on health, not all of which can be explained by the health risks associated with reductions in income.

Having helpful others in our lives enables us to keep feelings of catastrophe at bay and to strike a balance we feel comfortable with between dependence and independence. It is good for our health to have a place where we feel we belong in the social world. But having *intimate* others in our lives whom we esteem and by whom we feel loved involves an altogether more thorough-going sense of *our living through them* and *them living through us*. This conundrum is an old one in philosophy. Aristotle explores it in the chapters on friendship in his *Nicomachean Ethics*. The French philosopher Emmanuel Levinas, to take a more recent example, makes a sharp distinction between what pass for ordinary human relations, characterized by contractual reciprocity resulting in 'mere transfers of sentiment', and true human engagement, based on an encounter with the face of the other.[36] The encounter is always somewhat traumatic in Levinas's account because it wrenches us out of narcissistic self-sufficiency.

Winnicott said that holding always creates something new. No doubt he was thinking of the unfolding of the infant's capacities in response to early care. But the care of sick adults also offers a striking illustration of this point. It is not unknown for a condition to become as much a part of the carer's identity as it is of the person they look after. This can often be seen clearly in the case of the parents of children with Down's Syndrome who describe how enriching life with a Down's child can be. This aspect of holding environments was well captured by the philosopher Paul Ricoeur when he remarked that care is a crucial motivator in 'the search for equality in the midst of inequality'.[37] The pursuit of equality (or, in the case of parents and children, equity), potentially over quite a long period of time, comes to displace contractual obligations.

Holding in adult life doesn't have to have the intensity required for rearing small children. Winnicott once said that the family is best seen as a 'simplified version of society, one which can be used for the purposes of essential emotional growth, until development brings about in the child a capacity for using a wider circle, and indeed an ever-widening circle'.[38] This definition can easily be adapted to many intimate living arrangements. People routinely improvise simplified versions of society for those they love. Anyone who has participated in, or even witnessed, the care of a person suffering from dementia will be aware of this process. This versatility teaches us something that is often overlooked about the intimate sphere. One of its primary functions is to afford its members a degree of immunity from the demands and expectations of society at large. In optimal circumstances, a child will be able to use family life so that over time he can learn to identify with society without too great a sacrifice of his own individuality. But a person with dementia requires their individuality to be affirmed in a different way, often by having others remember who they were and what mattered to them.

In Chapter One we consider some of the ways in which illness activates the collective dimensions of human psychology, dimensions that highly individualistic societies like ours tend to minimize, if not ignore. These dimensions become conspicuous when illnesses first emerge, either in the form of possible pathognomonic signs or just after a diagnosis is made public. Our first recourse in the face of pathognomonic signs is to normalize them by treating them as transient aberrations.

After a major diagnosis, a process of group sorting usually takes place. We ask 'Am I a *friend* of this person? What sort of friend?

A close friend or a more distant one? Where do I come in X's pecking order? Y is a closer friend to X than I am. If I visited a sick colleague, might he feel I was intruding on his or her privacy?' Again, it is important to bear in mind that the answer to that question might well be yes. Illness is stressful and individuals vary in the degree to which they need time alone in which to process it. Nevertheless, over time, illness compels all parties to make visible who is in the intimate sphere and who wishes for more distance. Who will be in the holding environment and who will be in interaction order? And who will withdraw altogether? Illness shows us how rule-bound our social relationships really are. These are often more inflexible than we expect them to be, and it is when illness is just emerging that this first becomes apparent. To many ill people it comes as a great shock.

It is at this point that our study of the collective psychobiological dimensions of illness begins. We begin by outlining and extending Winnicott's ideas on holding. In holding relationships, we note, there is a partial pooling of psychophysical resources; this results in the healthy not noticing signs of emerging illness in a close other, or – just as striking after a diagnosis – a very powerful identification with their condition. Among intimates, the normalization of symptoms usually serves to sustain the pooling of resources. Among non-intimates, the situation is more complicated.

Once the presence of an illness is acknowledged, there are, we believe, only two major courses of action open to healthy others: they can either draw closer to the sick other, or they can abandon him or her (perhaps on the assumption that others will step in).

Drawing closer, the subject of Chapter Two, has its own logic or trajectory: it culminates, we suggest, in *care*. Drawing closer often rests upon two or more people being in deep, nonverbal, often unconscious partnership with one another. Using infant research as our model, we describe how humans draw closer to one another in normal, healthy life before considering the impact illness has on these habitual techniques. Here we draw especially on the work of contemporary infant researchers such as Colwyn Trevarthen, Edward Z. Tronick, Daniel N. Stern, Beatrice Beebe and others.

There are two basic ways of drawing closer to another person, corresponding to the two modes of intersubjectivity described above. Winnicott and his successors in infant research teach us about the richer mode, the one that culminates in care. But Goffman teaches us about more conditional forms of coming together based on attunement to the movements of others. It often happens that relations between the healthy and the sick come to grief because the latter want to be 'held' but find they are offered something more restrictive.

When the term 'care' is used in connection with health, it usually refers to an intersubjectively driven, potentially open-ended, practical response to a call for help arising from some impairment or loss of function. It does not always require a high level of engagement on the part of the clinician. Infant research construes care rather differently. It sees it as the effort to enhance the self-organizing capacities of a needy other by forming a synergistic system with them. We think the infant researchers' model of care tells us a great deal about how medical care actually works and in the course of this chapter, we make this case in detail.

In Chapter Three we turn to care's opposite, 'the pariah syndrome'. The pariah syndrome, as we see it, is merely the most extreme expression of the abandonment with which all ill people are threatened. Abandonment, in our view, is not just a possibility in the societies of the affluent West, but a strong probability. Our discussion unfolds in three parts. In the first, we draw attention to the biological strengths that groups of healthy humans can offer one another in the face of adversity. One of the most important of these is the building up of shared autonomic resilience, which enables the individual to harness the physiological power of the group. We argue that many Western societies are set up in such a way that it is harder for the individual to draw upon these strengths. Crucially, this affects those who might support a sick person as much as the person with the illness, and the consequences are often devastating. In the second part, we develop this theme by considering the ways in which healthy individuals typically help one another to cope with a strangeness that is intrinsic to ordinary embodiment and survey some of the ways in which illness might obstruct or inhibit those processes. Drawing on the ideas of a range of critical phenomenologists (Frantz Fanon, Iris Marion Young, Gayle Weiss, Bernhard Waldenfels), theorists of therapeutic change (notably the members of the Boston Change Process Study Group) and social neuroscientists such as Stephen W. Porges, we suggest that the expectations of the healthy in these matters are more stringent than most healthy people allow themselves to know and more apt to go awry in the presence of bodily dysfunction. These altered expectations explain some of the incomprehension that can take root very suddenly once illness enters the picture in relationships that were previously stable.

Finally in this chapter, we turn to the related question of the impact of this phase of modernity on how most people think about and indeed live out our notions of health, the body and death. We argue that what the sociologist Helen Fein memorably called the 'universe of obligation' – 'the circle of individuals and groups toward whom obligations are owed, to whom rules apply, and whose injuries call for amends' – has for most people in Western societies become smaller and more plastic. This, as much as anything else, explains why the social networks of the ill often become so much thinner. Towards the end of the chapter we consider three specific features of contemporary modernity that complicate relations between the healthy and the ill in ways in developed societies. These concern the assumptions habitually made in them about health, the body and death. We demonstrate that it is the *idea* of illness more than its reality that drives the healthy and the able-bodied away, which is why those with invisible conditions are just as likely to be turned into pariahs as people with visible conditions. We conclude with a critique of evolutionary-psychological accounts of the pariah syndrome.

The behaviours of distancing and drawing nearer at the heart of our account of shared life have a larger context. They are, as we demonstrate in Chapter Four, what George Engel would have called biopsychosocial behaviours or what Nancy Krieger would call ecosocial behaviours. Biopsychosocial approaches attempt to explain the fact that we flourish or decline in response to distinctive interacting biological and psychosocial stressors and buffers (anti-stressors) in our environment. This is in contrast to biomedicine, which only considers biological defects and insults. Drawing nearer and pulling away are characterized by distinctive physiological states whose contrasting biological content can be described in sufficient detail to make the difference between them clear. Drawing nearer, as we saw, involves *actively* suppressing the sympathetic nervous system. It means inhabiting 'one mind-time and one body-related space' with another person – a formidable set of demands by itself – and requires us not only to engage in neurobiological coregulation with another person but to become intimately involved in a kind of dance of movements, sounds and affects with them. Some degree of subject–object confusion is intrinsic to the whole process.

By contrast, pulling away enables us to escape all these entanglements. But escape comes at a price, namely that of cutting ourselves off from the supportive biopsychosocial resources in the group, most significantly the group's capacity to foster in all its members a threshold of collective neurobiological synchrony that buffers it against the adversity that is so hazardous for the body and the mind. This will be the case regardless of who pulls away, whether they are healthy or ill.

In ordinary, healthy life, isolation has been shown to be bad for human health over the longer term while support has been shown to be good. This, in highly condensed form, is the chief finding of a range of studies in epidemiology, epigenetics and social neuroscience completed since the 1980s. The absence of care, as we construe it in Chapter Two, seems to be associated with higher incidences of cancer, heart disease, stroke, diabetes and a variety of psychiatric disorders. Its presence is correlated with a longer, healthier life. Among clinical professionals, this evidence is widely seen as lending support to biopsychosocial approaches to health and disease.

We suggest that living organisms necessarily have a 'point of view' on their environment which guides how they construct their world. This point of view has to be narrativized at some level if we are to identify with our own 'agentive selves'. When our narrative purchase on the world is invalidated, when we cannot measure up to our culture's notions of what an agentive self should be, we become unwell. We lose some or all of the buffering that comes with social belonging. These theoretical additions enable us to articulate a biopsychosocial theory of resilience.

The Conclusion draws the major threads of this book together and explores some of the implications of the argument we have been making. All of the theories we have drawn upon in this book are rooted in what is now called relational ontology. They all try to explain what it means to be human by considering the many different ways in which humans are constituted in relationship with one another. They all see the relations as having a kind of ontological priority over the entities themselves. And finally, the relatedness with which they are concerned is often not directly cognizable in real time. This leads us to stress the importance of unconscious phenomena in human affairs in general but in this area in particular. Most of the Conclusion is devoted to disentangling the many different kinds of unconsciousness with which we have been concerned in this book.

We stress the importance of systems theory and systems biology for the future of the medical humanities and we end with a series of practical suggestions to keep the healthy and the sick able to relate to one another in mutually rewarding ways.

1

Emergent Illness

Illness is an instance of what some social anthropologists call 'trouble'.[1] 'Trouble' is a generic term that refers to any disturbance to the life of a group. The term is deliberately vague, because it attempts to capture both the ubiquity of such disturbances and the fact that they come in so many different guises: failure of the harvest, social conflict, imprisonment, endogenous shocks of various kinds. One of the most important functions of groups is to reassure us that our troubles are transient and that, in the event that they should prove more lasting, we will not be left alone. If I say 'I feel unwell', I am implicitly asking for others' sympathy, support and reassurance that my complaint can be tolerated by the group. It is usually in the group's interest to give me those things because doing so is likely to make the trouble I embody less conspicuous. It also keeps up group morale by giving the group an opportunity to demonstrate its power concretely. Symptoms are, among other things, requests for help.[2]

The same anthropologists tell us that trouble is typically dealt with by 'normalization'. Normalization is based on the assumption that the new reality can be incorporated into the old reality. It is an effort to affirm the validity of a pre-existing state of affairs, insofar as the new situation allows. When we confront a disturbance as trouble, we are holding fast to the pre-existing state of affairs. What counts as trouble depends in part on the modes of normalization available in any given situation. If I say I've got chest pains, you might suggest I see a physician. Alternatively, you might urge me to make my peace with God. Normalization depends on modes of acting and thinking that make sense culturally. It always involves multiple negotiations. In the illness case, these might involve concepts (for example: what counts as an illness in a given culture?), social realities (how will it affect the way others see me and act in relation to me? What sort of support can I expect?) and even bodily states (will my friends want to go on knowing me if my appearance deteriorates or if my voice changes?). In fact, at every stage of the illness process, there is scope for negotiation, not only by the person seeking to have his illness recognized but by those from whom he seeks recognition. The possibility that such recognition could be withheld brings us up against one of the central but often-overlooked facts about illness: we need others' permission to be ill. It is when normalization fails that intimate others tend to move closer while people in the middle distance pull away. Stigma, in many respects normalization's opposite, then rears its head.

In WEIRD societies, we are used to thinking about the individual as the most important locus of action in all matters pertaining to health. But in fact, the more closely you look at how individuals respond to signs of emergent illness, in themselves or in others, the more striking the effect of group belonging seems to be. Take diagnosis, for example. It seems natural to suppose that symptoms are what impel the individual to seek medical help. This is at best half true. It depends on the symptom and what we believe it heralds. As the medical sociologist David Mechanic has observed, in the course of growing up, most of us assimilate a selective version of the medical model and learn how to respond appropriately to common complaints.[3] The symptoms for which patients are most likely to consult a doctor are those for which they think a prescription will be helpful or those that appear to leave us with no immediate choice, such as the chest pains announcing a heart attack. Surprisingly, we are much more hesitant about consulting a doctor for other serious conditions. In an online survey of 1,724 adults in England carried out by the British market research company Populus in the summer of 2018, 48 per cent of respondents said they would not consult a doctor straight away if they experienced a symptom they believed indicated cancer.[4] In considering whether to consult a doctor, the most decisive consideration is whether the symptom interferes with the patient's job or personal life. In one of the classic papers of medical sociology, 'Pathways to the Doctor: From Person to Patient' (1973), Irving Zola and his colleagues found, contrary to expectations, that the decision to consult a doctor was taken most commonly because of a breakdown in the patient's family or other network's accommodation to the symptom.[5] They identified five triggers that led people to seek medical help: (1) the occurrence of an interpersonal crisis; (2) the *perceived* interference of a symptom with social or personal relations, that is to say, the problem was other people noticing it; (3) sanctioning ('I came here because my spouse said I had to'); (4) the *perceived* interference with vocational or physical activity; and (5) a kind of 'temporalizing of symptomatology' ('I passed out a week ago and put it down to tiredness but when it happened a second time, I knew I had to consult a doctor'). A UK study from the 1980s found that approximately eleven 'lay' consultations took place before a visit to the GP. These usually involved spouses or close friends.[6]

The fieldwork for Zola's study was carried out in Boston in the 1960s and we might expect it to have little or no relevance in Europe today. But Zola's paper remains highly cited and has been replicated by other studies in other parts of the world. A recent review of the most important papers in health psychology over the last fifty years identifies it as one of the first papers to demonstrate how '[culture] and social networks shape habits and behavior in [*sic*] almost an unconscious level, having a strong impact on how we cope with stress and handle anxiety.'[7] And the core finding remains true. A study of consultations in the UK in 2007 found that 'Following the detection of a symptom, the majority of individuals do not seek professional help, but instead do nothing or self-medicate.'[8] These delays often result in unnecessary complications and cause considerable numbers of avoidable deaths.

Illness, then, shines a powerful light on our social networks, revealing all their strengths and weaknesses. In any situation where we fear that our social standing may be downgraded, it is natural to appeal to the standards of those we love and trust the most. Diagnoses are life-changing in part because they have the power to change how even close others see us. This is something every person with a major illness understands. Diagnoses also have the potential to transform the social identities of their loved ones. Healthy people's subliminal awareness of this often comes out in the form of gallows humour. The poet and essayist Anne Boyer reports a conversation with a colleague that occurred shortly after she was diagnosed with breast cancer:

> 'Promise when I am ill, you will take me out back and shoot me,' a person at work said. Sometimes people told me, 'I would rather die than ...' – the ellipsis to be filled in with how they would rather be dead than do what I must do to live.[9]

The barely concealed meaning of these quips is that death is genuinely heroic because it takes the group's interests into account, whereas soldiering on doesn't.

Genealogies of normalization

The primary function of normalization is to hold the group together by asserting that the future will be the same as the past. This conception goes back to the work of the Cambridge psychologist Frederic Bartlett's classic book *Remembering* (1932).[10] Bartlett argued that our whole mental life is coloured by certain 'predetermined reaction tendencies', chief among which is a wish to make sense of the present in terms of the past. When we perceive something, we try to make it conform to something we know. The same is true of remembering. Memories are coloured by a different set of predetermined reaction tendencies. Chief among these was 'the effort after meaning'. If Bartlett's subjects were asked to remember an unusual shape, they often did so by connecting it with something familiar. They might call it 'a backwards Z with a line through it', for example. Faced with a complex visual object, some tried to take in the whole image at a single glance; others were more cautious. Bartlett found that 'an attitude of hesitation or doubt could have a powerfully negative effect on performance.' If they had to memorize a complex sequence of shapes, subjects often fell back on impressions or feelings. They would say things like 'I have a *feeling* it was like this.' This gave rise to a third reaction tendency, the power of inference. 'We often project patterns where there are none because they conform to an idea we evolve.' Nowhere was this clearer than when he asked his subjects to remember a complex Native American folk tale called 'The War of the Ghosts', which they were then asked to recall at intervals of hours, days, weeks and months. Bartlett found that with each retelling, his subjects eliminated more of its unfamiliar elements and replaced them with more familiar ones. Canoes became boats, seal hunting became fishing and not infrequently the ghosts themselves disappeared and the story became one about a war between tribes. Bartlett realized that humans are perfectly capable of recognizing the new. But we do it, he suggests, contrary to a deep inclination. Bartlett traced this tendency to distort what we perceive to our evolutionary inheritance. If our primary advantage over other species stemmed from our ability to cooperate, then an ability to affirm the value of our way of life over any perceived threat to it would be adaptive because it would entitle us to a share in any fruits of cooperation. He concluded that we were destined to misrepresent the world before us for the sake of being in sync with our peers. It is adaptive for us much of the time to proclaim that '*our* reality is *my* reality.' In this way, everyone can believe that the future will be like the past, which Bartlett took to be the ultimate aim of normalization. Whatever obstacles strew our path now are transient deviations from a more powerful underlying trend that will sweep them away. Normalization has a highly constructive side because it enables us to retain intersubjective connections in times of difficulty. But it carries with it some of the disadvantages of automatic denial and groupthink. Our commitment to it nevertheless expresses an important truth about human life, namely that the survival of the group is more important than the survival of any of its individual members.

The philosopher-sociologist Harvey Sacks offered wonderful descriptions of the lengths to which human beings will go to hide their troubles, even from themselves, by normalizing them pre-emptively. In a famous lecture entitled 'On Doing "Being Ordinary"', Sacks pointed out how much energy humans sink into portraying themselves as normal. Sacks recounts an eyewitness recollection from a book about concentration-camp internees in the Second World War. The first hours of incarceration are horrifying. Then there is a lull. 'Little by little conversation sprang up from bunk to bunk.

The rumours were already beginning to circulate. Luckily, the news is good. We'll be home soon. We'll have an unusual experience to talk about.' Sacks finds the same process at work in first-hand accounts of being caught up in a plane hijacking:

> The latest one I happened to find goes something like this. I was walking up towards the front of the airplane and I saw the stewardess standing facing the cabin and a fellow standing with a gun in her back. And my first thought was he's showing her the gun, and then I realized that couldn't be, and then it turned out he was hijacking the plane.[11]

The moral Sacks drew from these anecdotes was striking. 'People monitor the scenes they are in for their storyable characteristics. And yet the awesome, overwhelming fact is that they come away with *no* storyable characteristics.' We soften down the rough edges of our experiences by presenting them merely as 'things we saw' or 'the sort of thing that could have happened to anyone'.

Sacks's account of how 'doing being ordinary' actually works has been widely taken up within disability studies. Consider this example from Irving Zola, whose essay 'Pathways to the Doctor' we discussed earlier. Zola's autoethnography, *Missing Pieces* (1982), describes how his largely successful attempt to live a life as a 'normal professor' required him to hide aspects of his disability *from himself*. Zola had had polio as a child and was badly injured in a car accident when he was nineteen. Consequently, he had to have a steel implant surgically inserted into one of his legs and walked with a limp. One day in the late 1970s, he fractured his heel and went to work on crutches. To his amazement, none of his colleagues asked him what had happened. He seethed and finally confronted a friend who told him:

'Well, Irv, I really didn't want to upset you. I didn't exactly remember what you had, but I thought it was some kind of chronic disease and you were now in some kind of downward phase.' It was then that I realized how alienated I had become from my own condition. Not only did my friends reinforce this separation but so did I. The separation was so great that only a few friends knew the facts of my auto accident and polio and fewer still, the history that went with them. They never asked and I never told them.[12]

The formulation 'some kind of chronic disease' is a wonderful instance of illness as trouble: an ill-focused threat to ordinary life. In order to be perceived as a normal person, Zola had driven his disability to the margins of his identity. He believed that there was no shared language that would enable the healthy and the able-bodied to understand what it was like to be only partly autonomous. The 'core problem', according to Zola, was this:

> The teller finds it especially hard to acknowledge the central difficulty. Even to think about the world in such a realistic, paranoid way might make it too depressing a reality to tolerate. The only defence, the only way to live, is to deny the reality. But then it becomes socially invisible to *all* . . . Both those with physical handicaps and those without – *all* – are deprived of the knowledge, skills, resources, and motivation necessary to promote change.[13]

After this episode, Zola resolved to make his disability more visible and to ask for help. He used a wheelchair for long-distance travel and refused to give lectures in halls that weren't completely accessible. This is just one of the ways in which normalization restricts the life of those with disabilities. Most of the problems that disabled activists have described as problems of disability apply to sickness too. People with chronic illnesses often find they are put under great pressure to deny the effects of their condition. Chronic pain patients in particular have written extensively about the imperative to be silent when they feel like screaming, for fear of the effect it might have on those they rely on. This is silence in the service of what micro-sociologists would call 'passing'. It is also evidence of what Robert McRuer memorably called 'compulsory able-bodiedness'.[14]

In cases of illness, silence is the royal road to normalization, as a means of minimizing stigma. 'My mother's response to my congenital disability,' writes disability theorist Rosemarie Garland-Thomson, 'was to normalize it by ignoring it as fully as possible. When I talk about growing up disabled with other disabled colleagues, this astonishing family strategy for raising disabled children is their family story as well.'[15] 'A key rule for being a successful sick person is: Don't complain! The person who smiles and jokes while in obvious physical misery is honored by all.'[16] This was the most important advice Robert Murphy offered his readers in his classic memoir of a benign spinal tumour, The Body Silent (1987).

It should not be forgotten that the world offers chronically ill people powerful incentives to appear to ignore their conditions. In his book The Illness Narratives (1988) Harvard psychiatrist and anthropologist Arthur Kleinman relates the case history of a 46-year-old woman whom he calls Alice Alcott.[17] Alice was diagnosed with type 1 diabetes at the age of ten and had been taking insulin until the moment she saw Kleinman for a psychiatric assessment. Like many diabetics, Alice also had cardiovascular disease. Within the limits imposed by these conditions, she had led a happy and successful life.

Despite her condition, she gave birth to two healthy children who were now grown up. She loved the outdoors and led an exceptionally active life. But diabetic retinopathy meant she was beginning to go blind. Because she took pleasure in leading as normal a life as possible, she put off going to see her doctor until the symptoms were well advanced. One of her toes became gangrenous because of another delay in seeking care. Eventually the lower half of one of her legs had to be amputated. Kleinman is brilliant at describing the pressure to deny symptoms that patients with chronic illnesses like Alice and their carers suffer. Many of Alice's friends had no idea how serious her diabetes was because she had managed to make it almost invisible to them. Some might say that Alice's lifestyle was incompatible with her illness. We would prefer to say that her lifeworld could not embrace her body as it really was because the processes of normalization that lifeworld relied upon sought to make symptoms invisible.

Health psychologists Bruce Link and Jo Phelan argue that stigma usually takes one of three forms: keeping people in, away or down.[18] 'Keeping people in' is very connected with normalization because it is all about controlled inclusion. It allows the stigmatized to be admitted to life's feast on condition that they do not disturb it unduly. The afflicted should count their blessings. The depressed should pull themselves together, the psychotic should keep their more esoteric opinions to themselves and people with disabilities shouldn't dwell on them wearisomely. All of the examples we have looked at so far fall into this category.

'Keeping people in' can sometimes assume forms that are little short of unhinged. The sick person may find he is accorded a special place in the world as the bearer of, or witness to, some cosmic secret. When the blind theologian John M. Hull nearly walked into a car that was parked on the pavement, he was led around it by a man who spoke in a Middle Eastern accent. The man told Hull that his brother was 'badly ill. Badly hurt. In his car.' When Hull asked the man if he was injured himself, he replied 'No. This thing has never happened to me because I always look after people like you.' Hull remarks:

> He seemed to have greeted my arrival, around the corner just at that moment, as a sort of signal from heaven. It was a warning to him. These things had never happened to him because he always looked after people like me. I was a providential note, sounding in his conscience. I appeared around the corner with my white cane, just as his brother's car was coming to rest on the pavement.[19]

Hull's memoir is full of anecdotes about the ways in which his blindness turned him into a magnet for magical thinking by the healthy and the able-bodied.

The American disability activist Eli Clare, who has cerebral palsy, goes further and observes that illness and disability are often turbo-charged by other forms of discriminatory normalization. This vignette makes the point clearly:

> Strangers pat me on the head. They whisper platitudes in my ear, clichés about courage and inspiration. They enthuse about how remarkable I am. They declare me special. Not long ago, a white woman, wearing dream-catcher earrings and a fringed leather tunic with a medicine wheel painted on its back, grabbed me in a bear hug. She told me that I, like all people who tremor, was a natural shaman. Yes, a shaman! In that split second, racism and ableism tumbled into each other yet again, the entitlement that leads white

people to co-opt Indigenous spiritualities tangling into the ableist stereotypes that bestow disabled people with spiritual qualities. She whispered in my ear that if I were trained, I could become a great healer, directing me never to forget my specialness. Oh, how *special* disabled people are: we have *special* education, *special* needs, *special* spiritual abilities. That word drips condescension. It's no better than being defective.[20]

Clare's book is written explicitly from the point of view of someone who does not wish to be 'normalized' even under the licence of being exceptional. He sees normalization everywhere. In matters relating to bodily impairment, normalization underpins the ideology of 'cure'. Clare defends the rights of disabled people to seek cure but invites them to do so in a way that recognizes the shadow side of normalization, which he thinks can be found not only in most forms of social oppression but in our attitude to the environment.

A huge subculture has grown up for those on the margins of normalization. The Internet has enabled this subculture to flourish. Anne Boyer encountered it for the first time after she was diagnosed with breast cancer and describes it brilliantly. Here is a snippet of her discussion:

cureyourowncancer.org which sells cannabis oils and $45 snapback hats with a help leaf logo and the phrase 'I kill cancer,' claims, 'Big Pharma lies to convince us that their so-called cancer "cures" work.' The description under the nine-minute-and-forty-four-second YouTube video 'The Cancer Hoax Explained' simply reads: 'The Medical Industry Kills You.'[21]

Organizations like cureyourowncancer.org enable the ill person to reject the stigma of failed normalization by redefining their community. The person wearing the snapback hat proclaiming cannabis as a cure for cancer identifies himself as someone who belongs to a group. He is saying that he is not alone. There are others who see him as a locus of action in his own right, so crucial for the appearance of normality, even if the price of self-assertion is denying the legitimacy of the medical system. These counter-normalizing subcultures do to excluders what excluders do to the sick. They also pre-emptively dismantle the tragic narrative that the healthy and the able-bodied are so ready to build up.

Norms and normalization have penetrated post-Enlightenment ways of thinking and perceiving to a degree that is almost unimaginable. It is like asking someone to notice the effect of nitrogen in the air. They would notice its absence easily enough – it's just part of the given world – but its presence is harder to compass because it's so all-pervasive. Georges Canguilhem, Michel Foucault and Ian Hacking are the most searching analysts of this historic shift.[22] They all argue that normative thinking took on fresh importance during the eighteenth century, when, in Hacking's words, 'the idea of human nature was displaced by a model of normal people with laws of dispersion.' This alteration was paralleled by a shift away from determinism in the natural sciences when 'a space was cleared for autonomous laws of chance. Chance made the world seem less capricious because it brought order out of chaos.'[23] Medicine played an essential part in this transformation. All of those systems were exploded by the early nineteenth century but the normalizing function of medicine remained. For, as the sociologist Zygmunt Bauman observed,

One can view the opposition between the *norm* of 'health' and the *abnormality* of a disease as a pattern-setting specimen of the large class of notions which combined into the modern image of the world and of the human vocation in the world; one can say then that modernity in general embodied the 'medical stance' towards reality – it 'medicalized' the world.[24]

Foucault's account of the nosographic systems of eighteenth-century medicine in *The Birth of the Clinic* brought to wide notice the effort to reduce all illness to a very small number of basic categories. Conditions that had hitherto appeared exotic and uniquely anomalous became distant cousins of everyday ailments.

Canguilhem, Foucault and Hacking argue that normative thinking represents a kind of ideological horizon bounding our mental vision and that a powerful effort of consciousness is required to go beyond it. But they concur that it can be done. Norms depend on social enforcement – a point that has special significance in this book. Any given norm can, in principle, be suspended or overridden provided the *social* conditions of life contain the necessary flexibility for more than one person to do so. This, arguably, is the founding insight of disability studies.

Canguilhem liked to say that illness is best seen as a transition from one normativity to another. A healthy person, for Canguilhem, defines his or her own normativity. A young person might ignore the chest pains that herald pneumonia because he or she is used to taking strenuous exercise on a regular basis. But an older, less fit person is likely to be more attentive. A person with an illness must institute new norms of life, norms that are compatible not only with the biological limitations imposed by the illness but with group life. 'The sick man', Canguilhem writes, 'is not abnormal because of the absence of a norm but because of his incapacity to be normative.'[25] When Zola highlighted his own disability, it enabled him to insist that his own normativity as a person with a disability should be taken seriously by the world of the able-bodied. Alice Alcott preferred to live according to the norms of her youth. Rosemarie Garland-Thomson was discouraged from imposing her own normativity on others.

If Canguilhem lays strong and refreshing emphasis on the creativity involved in responding to illness, Foucault was more pessimistic about the capacity or the willingness of the world of the normal to grant full status to the abnormal. In *Discipline and Punish* (first published in French in 1975), he suggested that prisons, hospitals and asylums were designed to confine the abnormal and organize 'disciplinary careers' for them.[26] But Foucault also suggested that the organization of disciplinary careers generated new kinds of social identity, what Hacking would afterwards term 'new ways of being a person'.[27] For instance, in his lectures at the Collège de France on 'psychiatric power', Foucault described the rise of hysteria as an outcome of a kind of arms race between mostly female patients and doctors seeking to expand the domain of psychiatry by encompassing aspects of personhood that would not previously have been seen as warranting medical attention (in this instance, female sexuality).[28] The tragic achievement of the hysteric was to change the distribution surrounding the norms of femaleness and of nervous disease, and by that means to alter both.

Bartlett was surely right that individuals use normalization to bind the group together and that this behaviour has deep roots in our evolutionary past, but what we can learn from Canguilhem, Foucault and Hacking is that humans still have enormous discretion over *how* we normalize. The work of normalization can take many forms. Modern life abounds in institutions that aim to normalize constructively and limit the sphere of illness. Welfare states, healthcare services and progressive employment laws all constitute relevant instances. In the UK and in many other countries, if your disability won't affect your performance, you can't lose your job because of it. Employers have to make 'reasonable adjustments' for a person with a disability who is offered a job, or to an existing employee, to make sure they can do the requirements of the job.[29] Your employer must keep details of your disability confidential unless you give consent. You are obliged to tell your employer about your disability only if it has the potential to endanger yourself or your co-workers, or if it could affect your ability to do the job. For example, if you have epilepsy and your job involves operating heavy machinery, you need to tell your employer. In all other cases, you don't have to disclose it when you take a job, but if you don't you may not be covered by, for example, a company pension scheme if the condition recurs or gets worse on the job. Here, a discriminatory norm is partially overridden by the introduction of more flexible social conditions of life in precisely the way that Canguilhem, Foucault and Hacking envisage. And again, we might say that the progressive programme of disability studies is contained in this special kind of collective action. We might call this a more expansive normalization in which the minority is offered a way back into the social space of the majority.

The widespread public support for expansive normalization has led some to suggest that stigma is increasingly a thing of the past. Arthur Frank argues that the rise of patient activism has dealt a heavy blow to stigma.[30] Not only do patients not hide their allegedly spoiled public identities any more, but some actively 'out' themselves as carriers of previously stigmatized identities, transforming social attitudes in the process. There is no doubt that real changes in public attitudes have come about towards HIV, some cancers and even some mental illnesses. But stigma involves more than repressive attitudes. The stigma the ill face is rarely meted out in anyone's name.

It expresses itself most often in the form of embarrassment and quiet shunning. In June 2017 Macmillan Cancer Support, a UK charity that provides support to people affected by cancer, launched a national campaign under the slogan 'A mate with cancer is still a mate.'[31] The very existence of the campaign pinpoints where the stigma of illness really lives: in that obscure territory between professional and family life. There is ample research evidence to support the claim that people affected by illness – intimate others as well as carers – continue to struggle with stigma. And Frank himself has called Erving Goffman's book on stigma 'perhaps the most useful of all sociology books to the ill themselves as they attempt to sort out their situation.'[32]

We agree with him that Goffman's book retains particular value. Most theorists of stigma today start off from some known prejudice and then consider the forms it takes in real life, either from the point of view of the person imposing the stigma or that of his victim. This approach has many merits. It has an invigorating moral purposiveness. It lends itself to the methods of the experimental social sciences. Controls can be used, statistics produced, and, by these means, stigma measured. As Ian Hacking has pointed out, there are no statistics in Goffman's work.[33] He proceeded in the manner of an inspired ethnographer, viewing stigma as an emergent property of the human attempt to form an intersubjective system with another person. In his theory, even the most harmonious interactions are shadowed by stigma, as a possibility overcome. His theory has the advantage of being exquisitely attuned to aspects of an interaction that fall short of stigma or are ambiguously stigmatizing in a way that more avowedly 'scientific' treatments often aren't. We will return to Goffman in Chapter Two.

For now, we merely note that it is possible for groups committed to a common vision simply to *decide* to ratify the other person's experience, regardless of any turbulence to which it gives rise. This is the mesmerizing possibility at the heart of all normalization. Such a decision can be seen in Barbara Rosenblum and Sandra Butler's *Cancer in Two Voices* (1991), which described their lived experience of Rosenblum's breast cancer, supported by a loyal retinue of fellow lesbian activists.[34] Barbara Rosenblum took the unusual but logical step of insisting she was being altruistic by giving other women the chance to care for her. 'I am only the first among our friends to have cancer. There will be others,' she wrote. 'I am trying to live self-consciously (and perhaps die self-consciously) in an exemplary manner.' Rosenblum is here introducing one of the master themes of our next chapter, on care, for she is saying that if it is given well, care benefits not only the person to whom it is directed but the person giving it. Hers is a perspective analogous to that of the feudal aristocracy, which recognizes that serving *it* can be a mechanism of civilization for society as a whole. She also introduces a possibility that troubled Talcott Parsons and many scholars writing in his wake, namely that illness can also be a source of joy, of liberation, of challenge, of purpose, of focus, as well as threat, for the caregiver if not always for the recipient of care. We are not far from the Catholic conception of illness as blessing, a conception modern industrial societies still find deeply disturbing but which surely has a renewed vigour as so many grasp for a more expansive normalization.

On 'holding' as a special form of normalization

The critic and novelist John Bayley tells the story of an Irish monk who wrote to Iris Murdoch, Bayley's wife, to ask if he could pay her a brief visit on his way to pick up a fellow monk from Oxford.[35] Murdoch and the monk had been corresponding by letter for some time, though by the time the request was made, Bayley had had to take over from his wife. On his arrival, the monk told his hosts that the Duchess of Abercorn had sent them her love. This was 'momentarily discomposing' – Bayley and Murdoch had no memory of the duchess – but things got onto a better footing once Murdoch and the monk sat down together. 'They became extraordinarily animated – she starting sentences, or ending them – he appearing to know at once what she wanted to ask, and filling the words they were failing to make with a professional abundance of loving kindness.' The monk told Murdoch his life story and talked of the special place her novels had occupied in his life and in the life of the Benedictine community in Glenstal Abbey, of which he was a member. He spoke with special enthusiasm of *The Good Apprentice* (1985) and *The Book and the Brotherhood* (1987), going so far as to suggest that these novels offered a blueprint for a flourishing monastic life. 'For the first time,' Bayley writes, 'Iris looked blank.'

> Perhaps she had detected a note of Irish hyperbole; perhaps she was simply puzzled about the names of her novels. What were they? From whom? But she didn't enquire, only asking for the third or fourth time. Where living? Where born? – and did he know Dublin?[36]

Shortly afterwards, the monk took his leave. Once he'd gone, Murdoch seemed pleased by the visit but couldn't remember much about it except that the visitor had been Irish. Bayley hints that this episode was a straw in the wind. He could see his wife's linguistic oddities and her failing short-term memory clearly enough, but he could not take the further step of considering whether she had a serious illness. He even insinuates that the monk had left them because he had understood what was afoot in a way that he as her husband could not: 'I felt he had taken my measure, not because he was a clever man but because his experience had taught him much about the stupidity of intellectuals, their obtuseness about the things that really mattered.'[37] Bayley himself did not register the fact that his wife had Alzheimer's disease until several months later, when the couple went on a lecture tour to Israel.

In the late 1980s, the writer and editor Sigrid Rausing was living alone in London studying for a PhD in the Department of Anthropology at UCL.[38] Her brother Hans had been addicted to heroin for five or six years and had passed through many rehab clinics. After being discharged from his latest clinic, his mother thought it would be a good idea for Hans to live with his sister for a while. They managed it for a few months but then Rausing asked him to leave. Hans had stopped washing and plates of uneaten food were accumulating in his bedroom. In retrospect, Rausing realized that her brother must have relapsed more or less as soon as he had moved in with her, but she could not see it at the time. This disowning of knowledge would occur many times over in the years that followed. In 2004, Hans came to visit her and fell ill after an enjoyable evening with their children. 'I feel sick, like Hans,' she wrote in her diary, thus avoiding the fact that Hans's sickness presaged something worse than a bout of unwellness.[39]

When the sociologist Albert Robillard was a graduate student at UCLA, he told his friend David Goode that while he was asleep he had kicked his wife out of bed. 'Later he shared that he had punched her once in the middle of the night as well. I remember thinking that Britt [the name by which Robillard was known to his friends] must have a lot of deeply repressed anger against his wife.'[40] In his memoir of his life with motor neurone disease, Robillard mentions these episodes.

He had experienced involuntary uncoordinated twitching in the legs – fasciculations as they are called – while in graduate school at UCLA in the 1970s and had them looked at by the school's neurology department. He was later told that these were almost certainly the prodromal symptoms of motor neurone disease.[41]

These anecdotes draw attention to some of the ways in which emergent illness is lived out among intimates, where pathognomonic signs are interpreted instead as temporary aberrations or as the disguised expression of someone's personality. The symptom is then allowed to fade into the background of everyday life. There is usually nothing amiss about this perceptual fading. It is an important part of how we manage ailments in daily life. Collective living leads us to respond to ills of all kinds as collective problems. Empathy is often enough to reconcile us to anomalies in a person's demeanour. The three examples all involve coordinated cognition of a peculiarly psychosomatic kind, where the distinction between the mental and the physical is handled in an intuitive, rather automatic, unreflective way to help sustain the optimism and security of the cooperating group.

One of the core claims we will make in this book is that we respond to signs of illness in close others in a completely different way from how we respond to the same signs in an acquaintance. As these three examples show, intimates tend to pool their psychophysical resources; this often results in the healthy not noticing signs of emerging illness in a close other, or – just as striking *after* a diagnosis – identifying completely with their condition. Among non-intimates, the situation is more complicated. They do not pool their psychophysical capacities to the same extent. There is less to defend and sustain when symptoms of illness occur. In consequence, they are often more alert to signs of emergent illness in others. Recognizing illness more easily, acquaintances have fewer defences against the emotions of unease and threat that accompany the recognition of illness. This difference is very fundamental.

In seeking to understand how this special form of normalization works in the intimate sphere, we have found Donald Winnicott's theory of 'holding' exceptionally illuminating. The theory we are about to present is an adapted version of Winnicott's theory. Winnicott was slow to apply to his theory of holding to ordinary adult relationships. The only place he did so was in a lecture he gave a few months before his death entitled 'Cure', written in 1970. The term 'holding' first appears in his landmark paper 'Mind and Its Relation to the Psyche-Soma' (1949/1953) and was further elaborated in his posthumously published, book-length case history *Holding and Interpretation* (begun in 1941, completed in 1955 but published only in 1986). Joel Kanter speculates that Winnicott may have been introduced to the term by his second wife, Clare, who used it in a paper on social work in 1955. The best and most succinct statement of Winnicott's own understanding of holding can be found in his paper 'The Theory of the Parent-Infant Relationship' (1960).[42]

Winnicott used the term to designate the manifold kinds of support that mothers offer infants and children. 'The holding environment', he writes, 'has as its main function the reduction to a minimum of impingements to which the infant must react with resultant annihilation.'[43] Mothers 'hold' their babies, not only by carrying them, feeding them and changing them, but by absorbing the mental states infants cannot tolerate by themselves. Winnicott liked to talk about 'the holding environment' or the 'facilitating environment' to emphasize the fact that holding depends on many contingencies and many actors. Winnicott says that a 'mother is able to fulfil this role if she feels secure; if she feels loved in her relation to the infant's father and to her family; and also feels accepted in the widening circles around the family which constitute society'.[44] The clear implication is that this love and acceptance also constitute holding at a higher level.

In what he calls the holding phase, roughly equivalent to the first year of life, 'physiology and psychology have not yet become distinct, or are only in the process of doing so.'[45] The infant nevertheless takes his first steps towards independence. He learns to 'keep alive the idea of the mother and also of the childcare to which he or she is accustomed, to keep alive this idea for a certain length of time, perhaps 10 minutes, perhaps an hour, perhaps longer'.[46] He also becomes more integrated. This is partly a matter of the development of his nervous system but it also depends on certain environmental conditions. If the holding environment is 'good enough' he will have 'more definite emotional or affective experiences, such as rage or the excitement of a feeding situation'.[47] His 'mind' will become distinct from his 'psyche'. Mind, for Winnicott, implies a reflective capacity; the psyche, on the other hand, is a term he uses for the body's reverberations in consciousness. The primary caregiver, usually the mother, makes a judgement about what the infant can manage and what he can't and supplies the difference. Winnicott thought it made no sense to talk about a baby independently of the holding environment because babies are so dependent on the care they receive. Hence his famous dictum that 'there is no such thing as a baby,' there is only a member of a nursing couple. Holding facilitates a gradual progress towards independence and towards integration but Winnicott took care to say that the infant must be allowed to regress to dependence and unintegration if that is what he needs to do. It doesn't mean that those achievements have been set to nought. Most adults will recognize that this need to be dependent and safely unintegrated from time to time continues into adolescence and beyond – but that is jumping ahead.

Among other characteristics of good holding, Winnicott lists these:

> Protects from physiological insult. Takes account . . . of
> the infant's lack of knowledge of the existence of anything
> other than the self. It includes the whole routine of care
> throughout the day and night . . . Holding includes especially
> the physical holding of the infant, which is a form of loving.[48]

If 'the ego is a bodily ego,' as Freud claimed, it is so only because it is underpinned by a two-person relationship in which the mother's body acts as a kind of prosthetic extension of the infant's. Or, as Winnicott puts it: 'This environmental provision is also a continuation of the tissue aliveness and the functional health which (for the infant) provides silent but vitally important ego support.'[49]

Winnicott took pains to say that infants will not feel 'held' all the time. Indeed, as the holding phase progresses and the infant develops a capacity to recognize his experiences as distinctly his own, he will be subject to 'anxiety associated with disintegration'. But in optimal circumstances he will have built up '*a continuity of being*. On the basis of this continuity of being the inherited potential gradually develops into an individual infant.'[50] In Winnicott's account, infant development contains its own forward momentum which can be interrupted and even set to nought if the infant has to react to 'environmental impingements': a very disturbed primary carer, for instance, or physical assault. If he is spared these misfortunes, he can develop a 'core self' and form real and authentic relationships with people on the basis of his own personality. He will not feel too overmatched by the world. The most important thing is that there should be no experience of catastrophe.[51] Catastrophe must be split off as far as possible. The second most important thing is that, consistent with his actual development, the infant should be allowed to feel independent and autonomous. In the holding phase, this is usually enhanced by the infant's eagerness to master new aspects of the world.[52]

Holding goes on beyond the holding phase. The child develops his sense of self by interacting in ever more creative ways with others who understand him and his limitations. Education has a strong holding dimension. A good teacher, like a good caregiver, removes a limitation on the child's capacity until the child can overcome the limitation himself. But in the early phases of holding, the child's capacities are extended in ways that do not require any immediate understanding on his part. He is allowed to assume that certain things just happen by themselves. We are dealing, then, in the first instance, not with Freud's repressed unconscious but with a situation in which the child is enabled to make use of a caregiver's mind as an ancillary to his own.

Holding begins as a form of symbiosis but, in order to function properly, the holding environment must also *let go*. Holding is all about timely differentiation. As Robert Kegan has put it,

> a holding environment is a tricky transitional culture, an evolutionary bridge, a context for crossing over. It fosters developmental transformation, or the process by which the whole ('how I am') becomes gradually a part ('how I was') of a new whole ('how I am now').[53]

Kegan observes that even though the holding environment must let go, the culture of embeddedness that it provides must remain in place as a sanctuary for the 'held' person to return to or as a point of reference against which to measure his own state of differentiation. He gives the example of parents allowing their teenage offspring to reject them for a time as a form of holding.

For most of us, holding does not end with childhood, because we go on parenting ourselves and because we do things for others – especially intimate others – in the course of maintaining relations with them. But holding takes related but different forms in adult life. Holding is essential in infancy but it generally takes place on a looser, more improvised and less visible scale in adult life. Still, if the sceptical reader will bear with us, we will try to explain why we think holding remains a conspicuous feature even of adult relationships.

It will be recalled that in infancy, holding involves two processes: maternal care and infant development. Winnicott says that when it goes well, maternal care is 'scarcely noticed'. If the infant perceives it at all, it is probably as 'a continuation of the physiological provision that characterizes the prenatal state'.[54] Caring relationships between adults also have a side that is scarcely noticed, and which is perhaps evident in John Bayley's acceptance of his wife's failing memory and in Sigrid Rausing's acquiescence in her brother's withdrawnness. This tacit support, we suggest, is the heir and counterpart to maternal care in adult relationships. It is the support we invite the other to take for granted. And, as our three examples show, it gives us an extra margin for living. Iris Murdoch can go on enjoying her status as a novelist (even though her novels are now only a dim memory to her), Hans Rausing can be tolerated as an uncommonly unsociable house guest and Albert Robillard can be left to address his unresolved anger towards his wife at some later date.

What, then, is the correlative of the forward momentum of infant development in adult holding relationships? We suggest that it lies in the possibility of thriving. The best adult holding relationships aspire to enable the other to thrive in some domain. This thriving need not be on a grand scale but there has to be some acknowledgement of, and ideally identification with, what the other seeks or would wish for. John Bayley knows that his wife Iris sees herself as a novelist. She might have been having an 'off' day when they were visited by the monk but he – and she – can take comfort in the thought that she will return to form soon. Sigrid Rausing has sufficient confidence that her brother has put drug-taking behind him to suggest that he find somewhere else to live. And David Goode is worried about his friend's capacity to thrive psychologically if he has to deal with so much repressed anger.

Christopher Bollas reminds us that in adult relationships there is also a third component of holding to be taken into account, namely the achieved self-holding of both parties arising from their having emerged out of childhood and adolescence.[55] This often surfaces in the form of dialogues with ourselves. We miss a train and worry we're going to be late for an appointment. 'No point worrying,' we say to ourselves. Most of us do this sort of holding fairly often. It takes place in silence, for the most part. As Bollas points out, it warrants the name 'holding' because in such situations we become responsive to our own projections and modify them as best we can. Like a mother with a baby, we make a calculation about what we can achieve by ourselves and what we need help to do. And we strive to do what we can within our own limitations.

It requires no great acumen to see that major illness will have a powerful impact on these three aspects of holding. The 'unnoticed', taken-for-granted aspect of care is pulled out of the shadows and suddenly becomes very conspicuous while the possibility of thriving darkens. At the same time, self-holding comes to assume paramount importance. It becomes the holding of last resort on which the sick and their loved ones are often thrown back. How well a person manages this may depend on *their* holding history.

The two most important functions of holding in childhood – to split off catastrophe and to extend the capabilities of the held person by enabling him or her to transcend dependence – are just as important in adult life. Nothing shows this more clearly than illness. When John Bayley observed his wife's failing memory but failed to consider whether she might have Alzheimer's, he was abiding by these fundamental norms of holding. He was splitting off catastrophe and giving her her independence. If he had seen his wife through the monk's eyes, he would have had to reckon not only with dementia but with the fact that her career as an author was almost certainly over. Added to this would have been the pain of knowing that she would soon be unable to recognize others or be recognized by them. He would also have had to come to terms with the changes in their relationship.

The same phenomena, we conjecture, were at work when Sigrid Rausing asked her brother to move out of her flat. She could see that he had stopped washing, that 'he stayed in his room like a neglected child, dirty and dishevelled' and thought he should leave only because 'he was not cleaning his room again, not doing the dishes, again'.[56] But the idea that he was taking heroin again did not cross her mind for some time. When Rausing felt 'sick, like Hans' she kept him within the community of those who are subject to banal everyday illness.

Rausing describes Hans's first admission to hospital and hints the clinical staff at the London Hospital may have known or suspected what was wrong with her brother but decided not to tell the family:

Why didn't I see it before that, when he came back from India in 1983? He was twenty. His hip bones jutted out, his upper arms were thinner than his wrists, he had cut his own hair. He was in hospital eating bagfuls of wine gums, hooked up to a drip. He had a stomach parasite, he claimed.

Perhaps he did.

The doctors and nurses looked on and said nothing.[57]

Prodded by her sister, she notes that the family had had no experience of addiction so had no reason to speculate. The splitting-off of catastrophe in adult life is very connected with denying death. The sociologist Zygmunt Bauman has suggested that in Western societies we deny death chiefly by giving one another permission not to look at mortality, our own or anyone else's. Serious illness disturbs this pact.[58] This surely explains a phenomenon we touched on in the Introduction, the 'premature widow syndrome', where care is taken *not* to ask a family member about a sick relative.

Having a 'good enough' holding environment is one of the sources of physical and moral strength for many people. We know this intuitively, but many people would struggle to explain why it works as it does. The other who holds me becomes a predictable other. If I hold him or her too, I become a predictable other. This is an excellent basis for cooperation. But that is only the beginning. There is a dividing line in human relationships beyond which our primary motivations are less selfish. On the far side of that line, primary motivations become, in fact, quite altruistic. It isn't that we put calculation in the relational sphere completely behind us. But it seems to be the case that the concrete steps we take in order to 'attune' to the other gives rise to a mysterious sense that we share our selfhood with him or her. Holding involves a deep merging of the self with the other so that we cannot always say where we end and the other begins. It is, we suggest, this merging that, in optimal circumstances, makes us feel truly strong. This is surely one of the reasons why the very existence of a reliable holding environment reduces our sense of dependence and increases our sense of autonomy. The distinction we are drawing here has a big overlap with the distinction used by many academic psychologists who differentiate between high- and low-engagement environments. Those with whom our engagement is highest tend to be those in whom we invest the most emotional energy.

One of the oldest and best treatments of this distinction can be found in the chapters on friendship in Aristotle's *Nicomachean Ethics*.[59] Aristotle asserts that there are three grounds of friendship: utility, pleasure and virtue. From an English-speaker's point of view, the term friendship will perhaps be unsatisfactory as a translation of Aristotle's term *philiā*, which includes family relationships. Friendships based on utility and pleasure will be coloured by calculation. The person who pursues friendship for their sake must calculate as to the best way to secure personal advantage of whatever kind or pleasure. The person who pursues a virtuous friendship, by contrast, finds himself setting calculation aside. He becomes extraordinarily open to the other. The philosopher A. W. Price has described this openness in the following terms:

> *A* does not have to guess that *B* is a kindred spirit by [what Proust calls] 'one of those sympathies between men which, when they are not based upon physical attraction, are the only ones that are totally mysterious'; instead, he discovers that they share 'a single soul' through joining with *B* in deliberation and activity. Listening to *B*'s counsels, he finds that they articulate his own thoughts; observing *B*'s actions, he finds that they realize his own preferences. Many of these thoughts and preferences could not have been dictated to

B from the beginning: they only become apparent to *A* as *B* speaks and acts in ways that match them, so that *A* owes to *B* his awareness of the mentality to which *B* answers as a perfect partner. The same should be simultaneously true of *B* in relation to *A*: each reveals the mind of the other to him in a way that he could not have achieved on his own. It is through observing the other, who is more directly visible to him than he is himself, that each discovers himself.[60]

In other words, *A*'s self-interest merges with *B*'s to such a degree that calculation in relation to *B* no longer gives *A* what he most wants and the same is true of *B* in relation to *A*. The prototype for this process is surely to be found in the workings of the early holding environment. In the course of mirroring back to her child something about himself that he recognizes as being of value to her (and possibly others too), she enlarges his sense of himself and at the same time discovers something about herself. The same is true in reverse.

Winnicott would suggest, further, that this openness and mutuality can have a surprising physical dimension too. An unconscious process of physical adaptation to the other's psychosomatic normality can often be witnessed in families or between new friends. *A* may adopt *B*'s diet and eat at *B*'s preferred times, *B* may begin to talk like *A*, or dress like *A*. If *A* says he doesn't feel well, *B* may wonder if there's something amiss with him too. This process of forming a single psychosomatic entity is perhaps the main reason why healthy family members and couples are often the last to notice signs of illness in one another. It goes almost without saying that a part of this process involves each party unconsciously lending his or her well-being to the other.

The psychosomatic dimension of holding sometimes surges to the fore in illness. Surprisingly often, carers fear they might have the same condition as the person with a major diagnosis. So commonplace is this phenomenon that in the UK, GPs are told to explore it in consultations. In some cases, of course, a carer might have good reason to fear they've got the same condition. The daughter or sister of a woman with breast cancer might worry that she's got it too because she's inherited some of her mother's genes. A dedicated smoker looking after a friend with lung cancer or coronary heart disease might be rattled by what they see. It also needs to be remembered that many illnesses involve generic symptoms – fatigue, aches and pains, and digestive problems, for example – which healthy people experience routinely.

However, when there is a sick person in the room these phenomena can assume a signal function. There is something about the power and intensity of being a carer that blurs the boundary between self and other. When Kathlyn Conway was diagnosed in her twenties with Hodgkins lymphoma, her husband David developed a lump on his neck identical in size and location to the swollen lymph node on Conway's neck. For a time, David kept the lump to himself but when it showed no sign of disappearing he felt obliged to tell his wife. A biopsy was carried out by the same surgeon who had operated on Conway. He established that the lump was in fact a protuberant muscle. David had twisted his neck so many times feeling for a lump that the muscle had become enlarged as if it were a tumour.[61] Such stories are common. If it is through observing the beloved other that we discover ourselves, as Aristotle contends, we should not be surprised to find it has a physical dimension.

We might also bear in mind the well-documented phenomenon in which medical students arriving on hospital wards for the first time believe they suffer from the same serious illnesses they treat patients for. This common occurrence was first studied in the 1960s when it was estimated that between 70 and 80 per cent of students suffered from it. At first, it was studied as a transient form of hypochondria but theorists of medical education today see it as normal. Brian Hodges writes that learning about a disease

> creates a mental schema or representation of the illness which includes the label of the illness and the symptoms associated with the condition. Once this representation is formed, symptoms or bodily sensations that the individual is currently experiencing which are consistent with the schema may be noticed, while inconsistent symptoms are ignored.[62]

Hodges leaves out the 'learning' prompted by the presence of a person's sick body. What all these phenomena show is the extent to which the healthy and the able-bodied unconsciously use other people's bodily experience as a template for their own. We do it all the time in health – usually without disturbing consequences. Once illness presents, this faculty becomes subject to an unusual challenge.

There are, however, a few characteristics of adult holding that are different both in kind and in degree from childhood holding. We have laid strong stress on the fact that all holding contains an element of mutuality. Mother and baby do something for one another. The mother extends her child's capacities and in return the child enables her to do something extraordinary for him. There is a sense that what they create together is unprecedented. This gives rise to a historical residue. Holding in adult life also includes a historic dimension that is less conspicuous in early life. For instance, it is commonplace for adults to seek out other adults to give them an understanding they were deprived of as children. Someone who grows up in a violent home may be grateful to find a partner who is temperamentally mild.

This kind of retrospective compensation is much more conspicuous in adult holding relationships. Of course, some deficits are never made good. This is crucial in understanding the 'good enough' adult holding environment because in health one of its functions is to contain 'unmourned losses'. As we shall see, major illness activates unmourned losses and these test the holding environment severely. By unmourned losses we are referring to undigested demoralizing experiences that have lasting effects on self-esteem. The term is in wide use among humanistic scholars of ageing who have observed how the onset of diseases of aging often exacerbate unmourned losses among the elderly.[63]

What do the healthy do with unmourned losses? Typically, they find a place for them in holding relationships. It is not a matter of entrusting these to the other so much as of 'parking' them with them. The other knows they're there. They won't pretend they don't know about them. Consider the hypothetical case of an elderly woman whose husband has recently been diagnosed with Alzheimer's. Her early life had been difficult. She was the daughter of a schizophrenic mother and had never been able to count on her own mental health, having suffered prolonged depressions. Throughout their long and complicated marriage, she has waited for him to show some initiative in righting some of the wrongs of her life. The diagnosis is a sign that he is very unlikely to do so. At first she reacts with violence and then with resignation. The point of this story is to underline the fact that illness activates unmourned losses not only in the person with the illness, but in others in the holding environment. It may not be irrelevant to note here that long-term illness or disability doubles the chances of becoming a victim of domestic abuse in England and Wales, according to the *Crime Survey for England and Wales 2013/14*. A similar pattern has been reported in the United States and in Canada. As Julia Segal observes, physical illness appears to make attack more likely.[64]

One of the core functions of the holding environment during infancy is to sponsor what Winnicott calls 'transitional' experience. Transitional experience arises when the child feels sufficiently held by his environment that he can start to relate to himself as a person. It begins very early in life. A baby gets used to being sung to at bedtime, for instance, and hears the lullaby not only as an expectable thing but as a thing that enables him to be himself in a new way. He has a larger experience of himself and his world. Or let us imagine him sucking his thumb. Certainly, we *could* say he is hallucinating the breast or the nipple; Hanna Segal, the psychoanalytic theorist of symbolic thought, might say he is *symbolizing* it very concretely. But he is also having a very real experience of his thumb that both is and is not the nipple. Symbolism has many gradations. The satisfactions it envisages are not always those of the external world. The theory of transitional phenomena was an attempt to shine a light on this very subtle territory. Winnicott believed that the capacity for transitional experience marks the beginning of creative life. As the child gets older, he acquires a surer grasp of external reality but the path is lit up for him by what Winnicott calls 'subjective objects' – objects and preoccupations that have been imbued with a compelling sense of something that is both his and not his.

In the same way that he concluded towards the end of his life that holding persisted well into adulthood, Winnicott also came to believe that transitional experience continued to play a crucial part in many forms of adult creativity. In a late paper entitled 'The Location of Cultural Experience' (1967), he began to articulate a position developed fully only in his late paper 'Playing: A Theoretical Statement' (1971) based on the notion that play lies at the core of most forms of adult interaction – a position we will develop further in the next chapter.

Creative participation in a holding environment requires a capacity to share an experience with another person, even if the other person's version of it is different from one's own. It also presupposes a capacity for joy in being alive. Elaine Scarry has written eloquently about how unremitting pain undermines and often destroys both these abilities.[65] This unhappy consequence comes about partly because the person in pain becomes absorbed in his bodily experience in a way that diminishes other commitments and partly because others lack the terms with which to understand what the person in pain is going through. The sociologist Richard Hilbert has said that patients with severe chronic pain 'are precariously and continuously approaching the amorphous frontier of non-membership' of the culture in which they live.[66] (The same is true of anyone with a condition that others suspect is not genuine.) In Winnicott's terms, the scope for a creative encounter between someone in pain and someone who is well is likely to dwindle. Pain, according to Scarry, deprives us of the possibility of 'world-making'.

This is not true of all illness experience. There can be great mutual satisfaction in rising to a difficult challenge. Harold Brodkey, in his account of his own slow death from AIDS, describes a marriage made much better by the nursing relationship. 'My arrogant deathliness', he writes, 'and her burning gentleness were dancing together in a New York light in our apartment. This was like childhood, a form of playing house.' Brodkey's wife, the novelist Ellen Schwamm, tells him that his illness is 'one of the happiest times of my life'.[67] In addition to cases like this one, we might also note that mystical experience often features in published accounts of major illness, especially if the illness is likely to be terminal. In his last television interview the playwright

Dennis Potter went into raptures over the blossom on the tree he could see from his study window: 'the whitest, frothiest, blossomest blossom that there ever could be'.[68] And in his own illness narrative, *At the Will of the Body* (1991), Arthur W. Frank often ends chapters with reflections such as this one: 'Where we see the face of beauty, we are in our proper place, and all becomes coherent. As I looked out the window it formed a kind of haiku for me'.[69]

For any kind of transitional experience to occur, it must be possible for us to stand in a different and more enriching relation to the world than we did a moment ago. Illness often makes that much harder for the well person. After her final bout of chemotherapy for ovarian cancer, the philosopher Gillian Rose went on a walking holiday in Wales with three friends, including her partner, whom she names 'Steve'.

> This time of greatest intimacy with Steve was also to be the last. In the half-week that he and I spent together after our two friends had left, he seemed marooned in a stilted affection, light-hearted and adventurous, and then discomfited, as if he were undergoing some esoteric ordeal of fellowship in which he was the initiate, I, the cipher.[70]

Steve left her not long afterwards. But such was the richness and inventiveness of Rose's own self-holding, she could write not one but two astonishingly creative memoirs in which she intertwines scenes from her life up until the time of her diagnosis with an account of her increasingly theologically inflected philosophy. Cosmological in scale, those memoirs are triumphs of transitional experience by any standard.

THREE FEATURES OF Winnicott's account of holding make it especially valuable to attempts to understand what illness does relationally. First, holding has a natural history in childhood and adolescence. Winnicott's theory enables us to understand the ongoing relevance of this developmental itinerary for adult life. Second, the mutuality and reciprocity that characterize holding assume peculiarly physiological as well as psychological forms. Winnicott's account of this physiological dimension explains why illness is often a blind spot among intimates. It belongs to his version of the unconscious. Finally, and most importantly, through his emphases on omnipotence as a condition of feeling well in the world, and on the relationship between transitional experience and bodily states of all kinds, Winnicott provides an excellent framework for reflecting on what holding makes possible, especially in the illness sphere.

All of the features of holding that we have discussed in this section are normalizing in the sense that they make adjustments that soften down or eliminate the effects of illness. Splitting off catastrophe and reducing dependence normalize in a very direct way. The containment of unmourned losses and the sponsorship of transitional experience are seldom described and go on largely invisibly. The creation of psychosomatic communities is something most people have experience of, without necessarily relating it to the support they obtain from others. Yet it is hugely important in shaping the relations between the sick and the healthy.

In the next two chapters we will show how these features of holding and holding environments are transformed once major illness enters the picture.

2

Care

The way care is given can reach the most hidden places
and give space for unexpected development.
CICELY SAUNDERS, 1996

In the last chapter, we considered how humans respond by default to emergent illness and we observed how difficult it can be for adult intimates to recognize the onset of serious illness in a close other. In this chapter we want to develop our picture of what major illness does to intersubjectivity by focusing on situations where illness is recognized. To that end, we consider the intersubjective dimensions of *care*. As we shall see, these both underpin holding and normalization and go beyond them. Following Arthur W. Kleinman, we start off from the idea that the practice of medicine is just one example of a much broader practice of care.[1] In order to situate medical care within this much broader practice, we want to give an account of the latter.

Care might be defined minimally as a positive orientation towards another in need. It must have arisen as an evolutionary necessity. If we are group animals designed to live as group animals, individual members of the group need to be able to look after one another. The power to cooperate – the capacity that shapes so many human abilities, including the capacity to reason – depends on being able to maintain a positive orientation to others, including others in need.[2] Care, of course, is just one way of cooperating with others. In an essay published in 2015, Kleinman observes that care has developmental roots:

> I think of care as first and foremost a developmental process that, whatever its biological basis, is learned and practised as part of personal development, social cultivation, and maturation of our sensibilities and capabilities. We learn to take care of ourselves and others. Our cares are made all the more real by the threats and vulnerabilities that affect people everywhere.[3]

On this view – which we share – care is a *general* human capacity that is developed in the course of growing up. It is a many-sided capacity, which means we do not all possess it to the same degree or in the same way. It is a capacity that can be professionalized, provided it has reached a certain point.

It would be absurd to make these points without acknowledging the depth with which they have been explored by feminists. The three ideas we have rehearsed so far – that care constitutes a broad set of practices, that it is a necessity for our species, and that it has developmental roots – have been elaborated in a variety of ways by writers as diverse in outlook as Carol Gilligan, Nel Noddings, Berenice Fisher, Joan C. Tronto and Virginia Held.[4] Within the medical humanities, Fisher's and Tronto's work has been most influential.[5] In what has come to be seen as a landmark article, they defined care as 'a species activity that includes everything we do to maintain, continue, and repair our world so that we may live in it as well as possible. That world includes our bodies, our selves, and our environment, all of which we seek to interweave in a complex, life-sustaining web.'[6] By calling care a 'species activity', Fisher and

Tronto intended to challenge the notion that care was somehow the peculiar responsibility of girls and women; the duty to make 'a life-sustaining web' fell on everyone. And by making 'our bodies, our selves, and our environment' the central objects of care, they expanded care's domain so that potentially at least it encompassed every facet of life. As Tronto herself has observed more recently, the concept is so broad, 'it seems as if almost everything we do touches upon care.' And she continues: 'Once we start to see caring, we will see it everywhere.'[7]

But feminist writers have generally avoided close study of the deep imperatives underpinning care. Gilligan's landmark book *In a Different Voice* (1982) engaged deeply with girls' development but its conclusions were controversial, especially among feminists;[8] more recently, she has argued that the ethics of care should engage with

> new evidence in the human sciences that as humans we are by nature empathic and responsive beings, hard-wired for cooperation. Rather than asking how do we gain the capacity to care, the questions become how do we come not to care; how do we lose the capacity for empathy and mutual understanding?[9]

These questions are central to the next chapter of this book.

Feminist thinking on care focused, naturally enough, on female experience. It had various starting points: for Gilligan and Noddings, the central question was how girls and women came to have a stronger awareness than boys of the relational dimension of human existence and the importance of honouring our interdependence; Fisher and Tronto were concerned with the social pressures determining who identifies care needs, prioritizes them, meets them and assesses the effects of caregiving in the real world. We will address a set of related concerns.

It is important to state from the outset that it forms no part of our case to deny that the work of care falls disproportionately on girls and women or that the capacity for care is powerfully responsive to socialization. Study after study shows incontrovertibly that this is the case. The same studies show that migrants, the poor and the elderly are more likely to find themselves in caring roles, paid or unpaid.[10] We recognize then that what might be termed the 'who-whom' questions surrounding care – who gets it? When, how and from whom? – are political questions requiring political reflection and political action.

Nevertheless, we want in this chapter to focus on something more psychological, what Kleinman has characterized as 'the intensity of interacting with another human being that animates being there for, and with, that person.'[11] This is a subject many caregivers have written about. Kleinman calls it 'presence':

> Presence is a calling forward or a stepping toward the other. It is active. It is looking into someone's eyes, placing your hand in solidarity on their arm, speaking to them directly and with authentic feeling. Presence is built out of listening intensely, indicating that the person and their story matter, and explaining carefully so that you are understood . . . Presence is drawn from within. Ordinary though it is, it can be exhilarating. The experience resonates between the protagonists. Here I am. I am ready. In this case, ready to witness, ready to respond to suffering. Here for you.

What Kleinman calls presence is arguably the central topic of Emmanuel Levinas's philosophy, although Levinas treats it in an ethical and even a theological light. For Levinas, there is no self without another to summon it to responsibility. We will be presenting a vision of relations between self and other that is more empirically grounded than Levinas's. We want to emphasize that this more psychological domain of care has a politics too, as the American sociologist Arlie Russell Hochschild's many books show.[12] Intersubjectivity can be and often is a vehicle for oppressive power relations.

Kleinman is surely right, however, that care cannot be understood without accounting for the kinds of intersubjectivity on which it depends. Something like 'presence' needs to be described in a range of situations, its limits circumscribed and its possibilities adumbrated. Most currently influential definitions of care take overt caring actions as their starting point (see for example Fisher and Tronto's 'everything we *do* to maintain, continue, and repair our world'; emphasis added). The list of caring actions is potentially infinite. Tronto breaks care down into four analytic phases: caring about (discerning a need in another); caring for (accepting responsibility to meet that need); caregiving (doing what you can to meet it practically); and monitoring how the care you gave was received. From our point of view, this sequence usually unfolds when a caregiver has already been primed to act caringly. We will proceed in this chapter in exactly the opposite direction by focusing as far as possible on a relatively small number of intersubjective precursors of caring actions. These are for the most part pre-reflective and often unconscious. All of the major feminist writers on care assume the existence of these precursors. Tronto, for instance, notes that 'care proceeds from meeting needs' and adds, rightly, that 'discerning a need is actually a complicated task.'[13] But the centrepiece of her analysis is constituted by the 'specific moral practices', rooted in deliberation, that go into meeting the need. It does not take account of the intersubjective 'static' that can get in the way of caregiving. Instead, it assumes a caregiver who can rise above that static.

We are not asking our reader to choose between the pre-reflective and the deliberative aspects of care. On the contrary, we need both if a coherent research agenda is to be developed around care. We need the pre-reflective to understand why so many caregiving relationships come to grief despite a degree of goodwill on either or both sides. It is also essential if we are to explain the diverse and far-reaching effects of care on caregivers as well as on care recipients. And it enables us to understand care in more complex developmental terms than a conventional social account. But we need the deliberative too if we are to get to grips with how the pre-reflective is acted upon and moulded in the social world. We also need it to override some of what we do by default and remake the world, as Tronto urges us, in a way that recognizes the advantages of interdependence over independence. And finally, we need both because with practice virtually everything we will describe under the rubric of the 'pre-reflective' can be made deliberative at least some of the time.

The model of care we will present comprises three main elements: mirroring, holding and compassion. We take the term 'mirroring' from the field of infant research. Infant research is arguably the richest field of research offering a window onto what might be called the 'deep structures' of human intersubjectivity. It describes in more detail than any other field the ways in which we rely on our bodies to relate to others. We will describe mirroring in detail in the next section of this chapter. It broadly refers to the set of processes by which two people indicate their awareness of one another. They make this awareness evident by *reflecting back* something they perceive in the other person. This process forms a bridge between two minds and – as we shall see – two bodies as well. Each person begins to inhabit what the infant researcher Colwyn Trevarthen calls 'one mind-time and one bodily-related space' with the other.[14] Mirroring is highly creative. As the Australian psychiatrist Russell Meares has pointed out, when a mother mirrors her child she 'gives back some part of what the baby is doing – but only some part and not all – and also gives him something of her own'.[15] In the intimate sphere, mirroring generally leads to holding in the sense outlined in Chapter One; that is, it allows the 'held' person to enlarge his consciousness and what Husserl memorably termed his 'sphere of ownness'.[16] Mirroring does not have to lead to holding in every case. Indeed, among non-intimates, it generally doesn't. The boundary separating mirroring from holding is subtle and is sometimes hard to discern. But, as we shall try to show later on, they each have a distinctive phenomenological 'feel', based on specific and particular expectations and rewards.

Mirroring and holding are the main intersubjective precursors of care. We might note in passing that mirroring is preceded by a decision to *recognize* another person. Arguably, it is the most primitive form of recognition. In the case of infants, recognition tends to occur automatically because carers are primed by evolution to recognize their offspring. For a variety of reasons, adults may wish to withhold recognition from others. This withholding always results in a denial of mirroring. The counterpart of recognition in holding is *ratification*: the baby sees his caregiver seeing him and vice versa. Ratification holds out the promise of future mirroring.

Mirroring and holding are psychobiological in nature and have their own natural history in every aspiring caregiver's life. They are the main intersubjective precursors of care and the difficulties they pose can be visceral.

The third term in our account of care is 'compassion'. We will use this term in the same way that it is used in the Anglo-American philosophy of medicine, to refer to the response to the other in distress. Compassion is understood primarily as behaviour; it is not understood in terms of feelings. We will pay particular attention to compassion as it manifests itself in healthcare. The behaviours we will identify with compassion grow out of mirroring and holding; they are a set of 'tweaks' or modifications designed to maximize the efficacy of clinical holding in relation to illness.

Throughout this chapter, we will be attempting to describe healthcare as a sphere of endeavour that is much more closely related to infant care than is generally understood. As we observed in the Introduction, healthcare is usually seen as an intersubjectively driven, potentially open-ended, practical response to some perceived impairment or deficit. The care of infants, by contrast, could be defined as the ongoing and prolonged effort to enhance the self-organizing capacities of a needy other by forming a synergistic system with them. The relevance of the second model to health can be seen from studies such as the adverse childhood experience (ACE) study led by Vincent J. Felitti and Robert F. Anda on behalf of Kaiser Permanente, which demonstrated the devastating consequences of childhood adversity on adult health.[17]

Infant research offers the most developed paradigm we have for understanding the forms of recognition we give one another by default. It tells us what we tend to seek from others and what we do with it when we find it. It also tells us much about the creative possibilities in mutual recognition. These possibilities are closely connected with care in the infant case, since without care they would not exist: an infant who seeks recognition is seeking care.

The counterintuitive thesis we will be defending in this chapter is that 'the logic of care' – to take up a phrase made famous by the Dutch philosopher-ethnographer Annemarie Mol – is intimately bound up with the logic of children's play because it involves a formidable amount of subject–object confusion: that is, the caregiver's experience becomes somewhat fused with that of the care recipient.[18] Human bodies and minds are designed to come together in certain predetermined ways that evolution by natural selection has primed us to seek from birth onwards. These ways turn on powerful elaborations of coordinated movement, arousal management and meaning-making. These combine to produce a momentum towards play, where play is understood as the pleasurable and creative use of the symbolic resources present in a relational context. The infantile pattern of care-seeking is in our view never fully superseded. Rather, as we shall attempt to show, as humans grow older it assumes increasingly sophisticated forms that allow dependence to be masked, the body to recede into the background of human relationships (except in very specific circumstances) and intersubjectivity to feel like something that is rooted mainly if not solely in acts of cognition. These disguises fall away once major illness strikes.

The chapter will unfold in four parts. In the first part we will describe mirroring and holding in the care of infants and their relation to coordinated movement, arousal management and meaning-making, paying particular attention to how these fuse to create a rich implicit sense of the self in the world. In the words of the infant researcher Colwyn Trevarthen, this gives the child a place in 'a community of "common sense", not just security in attachments'.[19] Through mirroring and holding, the child acquires a sense of belonging. In the second part, we demonstrate the continued relevance of mirroring in adult communications, drawing on Erving Goffman's notion of the 'interaction order'. We then turn to some of the specific difficulties that illness and disability pose for mirroring. Illness in other people, we suggest, is often experienced by the healthy and the able-bodied as a breakdown in mirroring (which in turn precludes holding). In the final section, we turn to consider professional healthcare. We argue that mirroring and holding are fundamental features of healthcare and that there is a far-reaching symmetry of means linking infant care to healthcare and to every other kind of care. But healthcare is also characterized by certain deontological behaviours which we identify with compassion. We argue that compassion is a response to some of the pressures resulting from mirroring and holding the sick. We conclude with a critique of Annemarie Mol's highly influential account of healthcare.

The care of infants

Paradoxically, the best way to understand what the care of infants tells us about care more generally is to home in on the very things that make it seem so unique. The most distinctive features of infant care arise from the extremity of the infant's dependence on the one hand and his capacity to become independent on the other. The caregiver supplies what the infant cannot manage by himself until such time as the latter's biological, physiological and mental abilities enable him to do what is needed for himself.

Humans seem to have an innate propensity to share the intentional states of others. Perhaps the most basic way they do this is by reacting to the movements of others. Daniel N. Stern and Giannis Kugiumutzakis have described experiments in which a grown-up sticks out her tongue or opens her mouth at a newborn and the infant reciprocates.[20] As Colwyn Trevarthen points out, the fact that this capacity is present in infants so young shows that it is subcortical, rooted in the most primitive parts of the brain, and involuntary. Only much later does it come under voluntary control and even among adults it remains partly involuntary. It is part of our phylogenetic inheritance as social animals. Infants do not consciously copy others; rather they discover that they *have* copied them through feeling and action. By the time they are eight weeks old, most babies can sustain eye contact with another person. Copying movements seems to enable infants to try out the other person's experience of the world for themselves. This is one of the ways in which they become attuned to the affective states of other people. The mirroring performed by infants begins with mimesis of movements but soon develops into affect attunement. The mirroring performed by primary caregivers goes beyond these by encompassing any form of what Meares terms 'responsive recognition'.[21]

In some respects, studies of caregiver–infant interactions echo the phenomenologist Husserl's suggestion that our capacity to understand the experiences of others depends on being able to simulate their experiences in our own bodies. An 'analogizing apprehension' of the other's body takes place.[22] Merleau-Ponty developed this claim by suggesting that we are obliged in a sense to 'pair' our experience with that of other people, much as you might pair two Bluetooth devices. 'In perceiving the other,' he wrote, 'my body and his are coupled, resulting in a sort of action which pairs them [*action à deux*]. This conduct which I am able only to see, I live somehow from a distance. I make it mine; I recover [*reprendre*] it or comprehend it.'[23] When we perceive the external signs of intentions in others, we do so by registering those intentions in our own bodies, as if they were our own, and, in this way, we create a context in which intentional states pass between ourselves and another. Merleau-Ponty called this context the shared body schema. Arguably, psychoanalytic theories of projection and introjection also rely on a theory like the shared body schema.[24]

By signalling that we are in sync with the movements of others, we develop a narrative of actions with them that forms the basis of shared meaning-making. Now it might be objected at this point that in the case of the baby we can't know that any such thing is happening because he is preverbal. But he can apprehend something of the moment-by-moment flow of the actions of those around him, of their internal states and his own internal states, and carers can pick up some of that response. These are the raw materials of shared narrative in infancy.

Entering these 'dyadic states', as Edward Z. Tronick calls them, is demanding for newborns because of the physiological costs of arousal to the very young body. Take eye contact.[25] Eye contact is a form of imitation but it is highly arousing. It causes the infant's heart rate to increase. Stress hormones are produced and the gut may be activated. Usually, after five or ten seconds, when the infant has had enough, he will avert his gaze and perhaps use his hands to screen his face as if to defend himself. The caregiver may try to restore contact by altering her position. Infant research suggests this is a mistake. The baby is trying to lower his own levels of physiological arousal. The more aroused he is, the longer it takes him to restore his own homeostatic balance. The way for the caregiver to repair the contact is to wait. If the baby perceives the caregiver senses his state – which she might show by moving back a little – he may use *her* adjustment to regulate *his* arousal. He may feel free to look around him. If her facial expression is less stimulating, he may begin to come back into the dyad.

Sequences such as this unfold over a period of ten or twenty seconds. They depend on micromovements that infant researchers capture using digital video equipment that enables them to break down each second of contact into sixty frames. These micromovements reflect psychobiological, affective, bodily based processes that are interactively regulated out of awareness.

Four points in our story so far should be noted. First, the infant uses two forms of regulation. He regulates himself by turning away from his caregiver but then he engages in coregulation with her when they recover a rhythm both can tolerate. Coregulation is a crucial invisible component of care throughout the life cycle, and we will come back to it at length in Chapter Three when we turn to adults.

Second, the move from alignment through misalignment to repair shows that humans learn to engage with and disengage from one another more or less simultaneously, on the basis of co-constructed and intermittently shared experiences. The German Marxist philosopher Ernst Bloch once observed that 'Shunning, isolating and detaching are just as much social acts as binding and uniting.'[26] Infant researchers would agree with him. Shunning, isolating and detaching are a fundamental part of infants' – and our species' – intersubjective repertoire. Over time, they give us a valuable measure of discretion in navigating the social world. There is a truth about intersubjectivity that is so basic it is easy to overlook. That truth is this: intersubjective links enable us to *do things* with others. For infants, shunning, isolating and detaching in the moment may be a way of saying 'I do not wish you to do anything with me now, perhaps because I would find it too arousing, so I've taken measures to make you disappear.'

Third, movement and rhythm are critical to the whole enterprise. Daniel Stern suggests that the mutual attunement of mother and baby is of the same order of complexity as the choreographing of a ballet.[27] They share a similar multimodal richness. A ballet marries music and dance and shape. A mother speaking 'motherese' to her baby might respond to a sound with a smile or a gesture, drawing on the multimodal system. Stephen Malloch and Colwyn Trevarthen have pointed to the 'communicative musicality' of carer–infant dyads.[28] Malloch and Trevarthen reported that the 'proto-conversations' of these dyads with infants as young as six weeks exhibit precise musical characteristics. They found 'graceful fluctuations in pitch creating a melody'. They also found that in addition to a regular beat and bar structure, a baby aged six to twelve weeks could participate in 'musical' interactions for around thirty seconds.[29] Each learns to orchestrate their contributions to a non-verbal conversation to produce predictable climaxes of affect. The underlying sense of rhythm may be enhanced by the baby's perceptions of movements. The baby who is trying to lower his own levels of physiological arousal uses movements – his own and those of his carer – as his guide. The micro-movements studied by infant researchers show that carer–infant dyads move in and out of synchrony. With practice and with the development of trust the synchrony takes the form of what Colwyn Trevarthen calls 'intersubjective motor control'.[30] Eventually, they inhabit 'one mind-time and one bodily-related space' together. Predictability is everything because it allows the infant to build up excitement and joyful pleasure. It is important to stress that caregivers do not have to be continuously attuned to infants: studies suggest such attunement occurs less than 30 per cent of the time.[31]

Fourth, mirroring turns on a reward system. In the case of infants, the rewards are dispensed progressively through the discovery of new possibilities in mirroring itself. The philosopher Jay Bernstein, who, like us, has been very influenced by infant research, puts the matter this way:

in the ongoing processes of mimetic responses – their increasing sophistication; their increasing real mutuality;

their sharing of pleasure in interactive success – there is borne and shaped in socially normative forms the worth of the partners to the interaction: child and parents become independent persons for one another. Hence, the mimetic dance is experienced by the child normatively as how she matters and expects to matter to others who matter to her; call this the mimetic dance of first love.[32]

All four of these points are illustrated in the universal phenomenon of childish play that is their natural point of culmination. Play involves being able to attune to the movements of others and to approximate their intentional states. It also increasingly involves dramatic wave-cycles of excitement. Winnicott, one of the shrewdest psychological theorists of play, offered the first truly compelling picture of the mother's or primary caregiver's role in orchestrating these wave cycles. Moreover, he saw her achieving this goal by mirroring her baby. In Winnicott's account, a baby invests his mother with meanings that come from himself; the mother then mirrors these meanings back to him; the baby uses this synchrony as a platform from which to consolidate this perception and then the process begins afresh. 'This means', Winnicott writes,

> that the mother (or part of mother) is in a 'to and fro' between being that which the baby has a capacity to find and (alternatively) being herself waiting to be found. If the mother can play this part over a length of time without admitting impediment (so to speak) then the baby has some experience of magical control, that is, experience of that which is called 'omnipotence' in the description of intrapsychic processes.[33]

Winnicott goes on to suggest that even when the infant learns to play alone, the caregiver – if she is 'good enough' – is felt to 'reflect back' what happens in the playing. In other words, the unconsciously internalized external object goes on mirroring even in her absence. In the final stage, 'the child learns to allow and enjoy the overlap of two play areas' and experiences pleasure based on 'the interplay of personal psychic reality and the experience of control of actual objects. This is the precariousness of magic itself, magic that arises in intimacy, in a relationship that is being found to be reliable.'[34] This talk of magic can be misleading. The thing we must never lose sight of is that what the child is manipulating are meanings. He is learning to elaborate the significance of the lifeworld.

Contemporary neurobiological accounts of play explain why these wave cycles are so critical in child development. Affect synchrony is widely seen as the earliest expression of social play.[35] In neurobiological terms, it is the arousing aspects of play that make it so beneficial to children's health and general development. Daniel Stern talked of infants needing to be '[blasted] into the next orbit of positive excitation'.[36] The intense pleasure infants take in play-based interactions with caregivers increases their dopaminergic arousal, which enables them to process novel information more easily. Allan Schore emphasizes the ways in which caregivers and infants' mutual recognition of each other's excitement reinforces their pleasure and the neurobiological substrate supporting it. At the same time, the soothing and calming moments in play are no less important because these take the rough edges off the infant's distress and reinforce his trust in the caregiving dyad. Here oxytocin is especially important.

For Tronick, the significance of dyadic states of consciousness is that they increase the coherence of the organism more generally.

In his account they have three characteristics. First, as noted, each individual's state of consciousness integrates essential elements from the other and as a consequence their state of consciousness becomes more coherent, complex, richer in meaning and more integrated. Second, there is an implicit and possibly explicit experience of knowing the other's state of mind. A psychoanalyst might say that the basis of their coming together at that moment is the mutual introjection of the other's state of mind. It is a moment of mutual ratification of one another's experience. Dyadic consciousness is not something that is established once and for all at the age of six or eight months. Rather, it is something that gets constructed in a variety of ways according to both parties' capacities. Finally, there is a powerful experience of becoming larger than oneself.[37] Dyadic states of consciousness bring mirroring to a point of culmination and initiate the process of holding we described in the last chapter.

Tronick suggests that infant minds are best seen as immature open biological systems along the lines of those described by the Belgian chemist Ilya Prigogine. In order to build themselves up, they have to undergo certain organizing experiences or else their living energies dissipate and they lose complexity and coherence as organisms.[38] In particular, they have to have an experience of others 'locking on' to their minds. Tronick is perhaps most famous as the originator of the Still Face experiment. In this experiment, a caregiver plays interactively with her one-year-old baby for a few minutes and is then asked to turn away briefly before facing the infant again with a still face. The caregiver is asked to maintain the still face for up to five minutes. Typically, most babies in the experiment dissolve into great distress within three minutes. In optimal circumstances, caregivers and infants regulate the functioning of each other's central nervous systems and autonomic nervous systems – cortisol levels fall, oxytocin rises, heart rates fall, respiration becomes more settled – and as a result, the infant's internal homeostasis develops. What the Still Face experiment shows is that without the scaffolding of the caregiver's mind, none of this can occur. In the next section of this chapter, we will suggest that the fact that dyadic states of consciousness are both psychological and biological can have a powerful effect on the quality of interactions between the healthy and the ill.

What infant research offers us is an object lesson in the inter-subjective precursors of care. It shows us that intersubjectivity is ultimately rooted in the coordination of bodily movements in time. This enables us to communicate with others either by direct imita-tion of *their* movements or by some other form of responsive recognition. Physiological arousal can constitute an impediment in the way of such communications. In a caregiver–infant dyad, this problem is typically addressed by sensitive recognition of the child's own developing capacities for engagement and disengagement and for self-regulation. It is these which eventually give him the ability to be an agent in his own right. Over time, the rhythmic coordination of movement leads to ever more sophisticated forms of mirroring, which ultimately bring about many different kinds of dyadic states of consciousness.

The infantile roots of adult communications

In considering how mirroring in general works between adults, it is well to keep in mind two broad rules of thumb. They are rough and ready; they are not laws, because they can be overridden at will by the parties to the interaction; but, as we hope to show, they are particularly enlightening when it comes to understanding why communications between the healthy and the sick so often go awry. The first is that humans tend to use others as mirrors in which they hope to find something of value in themselves reflected back. The second is that out of awareness humans ceaselessly scrutinize the implicit dimensions of interactional space in search not of recognition only but of the conditions that might support recognition.

It is important to point out that most adults have at their disposal a multimodal assortment of bodily signals as rich and as complex as any that can be found between caregivers and infants. Humans make their intentions, interests and emotions known to one another through bodily movements. By coordinating their movements, they orchestrate whatever vitality exists between them. The elements of this dialogue and the actions by which they are brought into synchrony with one another include metalanguage ('ums' and 'ahs', taking turns in conversation), rhythm, pitch, vocal cadence, the prosodic features of the face, movements of the limbs and general bodily demeanour (wariness or openness, for example). The experience of performing this 'dance' creates a sense of reciprocity.

Microsociology evolved a whole view of social interaction based on these implicit communications that, in the words of Harold Garfinkel, go 'seen but unnoticed'.[39] Perhaps the most comprehensive attempt to reclaim and resituate this bodily dialogue was made by Erving Goffman. Goffman was interested in how human beings interact in one another's presence. He called this face-to-face domain of group life 'the interaction order' and he spent most of his career defending it as an analytically viable category.[40] From our point of view, its interest lies in the fact that it offers an account of mirroring taking place between adults intersubjectively and on the basis of attunement to the movements of others. He also shows us that encounters in the interaction order turn on similar sorts of rewards that are in play in infancy.

In Goffman's account, the interaction order had an animal dimension that was somewhat resistant to the constraints imposed by social institutions (a claim many sociologists rejected).[41] In his final address to the American Sociological Association, he remarked that the 'the interaction order catches humans in just that angle of their existence that displays considerable overlap with the social life of other species.' This angle finds expression in the fact that we attune ourselves not only to the social markers others present – their dress, their accent, the social assumptions underpinning the relationship they attempt to strike up with us – but to the emotions they evince, their mood and posture. 'Ease and uneasiness, unselfconsciousness and wariness are central,' Goffman writes. Much of this is necessarily unconscious because it occurs so rapidly. The interaction order, in Goffman's account, was saturated with implicit knowledge that participants can barely articulate because it resides largely in the realm of the 'taken for granted'. For example, if we meet someone for the first time, we avoid staring at them. We make eye contact, if we can. We appraise the signals they give us in the knowledge that they are scrutinizing our performance no less diligently. In our terms, the interaction order functions largely through mirroring.[42]

Goffman's description of the interaction order took its cue from a description of religious life in one of Durkheim's most important books. In *Les formes élémentaires de la vie religieuse* (1912) Durkheim suggested that ritual is the glue that holds groups together.[43] A ritual might take the form of a religious service or a football game, say. The Eucharist is celebrated, a goal is scored, and the congregation or crowd expresses its emotional response to the symbolic meaning of these events as an overflow of powerful feeling. Note that there are three elements to the interaction. There is the ritual itself (the Eucharist, the football game) and the things symbolized by the ritual (salvation, winning a trophy) which together produce what Durkheim memorably termed in French 'effervescence collective'. Goffman transposed this framework so that it covered the most mundane encounters. *A* says to *B* 'Hi.' *B* says 'Hi' back. The ritual is saying hello, the symbols are the people themselves and their power to evoke meaning in the social world produces a glimmer of 'effervescence collective'. We might think of this effervescence as a sedimented version of Bernstein's 'mimetic dance that enables the neonate to discover how she matters to others who matter to her'.[44] The key fact to bear in mind is that for Goffman, as for the infant researchers, mirroring generates its own reward system. The rewards are biphasic. In the very short term, we enjoy the affirmation that comes from mutual recognition. This in turn leads to the assumption of reciprocity. The most rewarding and therefore the most valued forms of mirroring imply an intention to supply stable reciprocity.

It is still a precarious business. Merely by placing ourselves in the presence of another person, says Goffman, we make a promise to them about who we are. Our social self rests on this promise. The face we present to others, Goffman says, is 'a sacred thing' because it creates the social self. 'For a complete man to be expressed, individuals must hold hands in a chain of ceremony . . . While it may be true that the individual has a unique self all his own, evidence of this possession is thoroughly a product of joint ceremonial labour.'[45] But, of course, the threat of profanation hangs over both parties all the time. *A* may decide that *B* just isn't his sort of person and refuse to recognize *B* as another person at all. In such cases, if *B* wants to recognize *A*, *B*'s social self is discredited. His identity is spoiled. *A* too must seek a new interaction order in which his identity can be credited in ways he can value. If we are lucky, then, over time and as a result of multiple successful instances of mirroring, we will come to be seen as reliable.

'We lean on these anticipations that we have, transforming them into normative expectations, into righteously presented demands.'[46] The interaction order, like the social selves it sponsors, is therefore very fragile. The social self, Goffman writes, is 'a dramatic effect arising diffusely from a scene that is presented'.[47] This means that the social self cannot be taken for granted; rather, it has to be renewed constantly – a point to which we shall return.[48] Colwyn Trevarthen remarks that infants come into the world equipped with 'a talent for proud companionship in imaginative intentions for life'.[49] The pride they take in being included in the communal goings on around them connects them with a world of 'shared vitality experience, curiosity, [and] invention'.[50] We think that what is at stake in Goffman's interaction order is similar to the pride Trevarthen describes in his writings as being so crucial for healthy child development. And as we shall see, this pride is very important in relations with the ill.

Mirroring between sick and healthy adults

In casual interactions, what adults want first and foremost is for others to recognize them. In this limited sense, we are all egotists and opportunists. We are egotists because we need some token of interactive success that affirms our worth. In brief interactions with strangers, we are, as a rule, more interested in having our own worth affirmed than in affirming the other person's worth. This was something Arlie Hochschild discovered when she sat in on a training day for new airline stewardesses in the late 1970s, for her classic book *The Managed Heart*:

> The young trainee sitting next to me wrote on her notepad, 'Important to smile. Don't forget smile.' The admonition

came from the speaker in the front of the room, a crew-cut pilot in his early fifties, speaking in a Southern drawl: 'Now girls, I want you to go out there and really *smile*. Your smile is your biggest *asset*. I want you to go out there and use it. Smile. *Really* smile. Really *lay it on*.'[51]

The trainer, we may surmise, understood the purpose and importance of mirroring. Smiling not only promises stable mirroring, but suggests to the passengers that they will get more back than they will be required to give, which, as we shall see, is an essential feature of what some physicians term 'empathic witness'.[52]

Disabled individuals have shown us the astonishing extent to which the healthy and the able-bodied continue to rely on the silent dialogue of movements to navigate their way around the social world. The coordination of bodily signals creates a shared sense of 'real time' and a context in which to create peaks and troughs of attention with another person. When Albert Robillard was discharged from hospital, he could speak using a lip-reading translator, spelling out words letter by letter, which was necessarily very slow. He could barely move. He soon found that not being able to underscore his speech with movements resulted in social isolation. Robillard describes colleagues crossing the street to avoid having to greet him, strangers imputing idiocy to him on the basis of his wearing a bib, being abandoned at parties or finding someone had turned their back to him, blocking his frontal access to conversation, as if the guests at the party needed to be protected from him. Again, it is tempting to conjecture that unconsciously an assumption is made that the disabled person might pass his disability on to the other guests. As a paralysed man he could not illustrate his speech with the expected array of bodily actions: 'The essence of isolation, at least for me,' he writes, 'resides in the inability to indicate through my own bodily behaviour and speech the analysis of others' preceding and subsequent utterances and bodily behaviour.'[53] Others offered him no possibilities of 'intersubjective motor control'.

This suggests that, as a by-product of the most ordinary social contacts, healthy and able-bodied people supply for one another evidence of their rights to serve as partners in mirroring. Most of the time, these evidences are treated as mere reinforcers, peripheral to the central business of communication. But they are profoundly important in containing anxieties about our own status as worthy actors in the interaction order, which depends on having the ability to demonstrate normative knowledge of the body; that is, a knowledge of and commitment to how the body *should* be. Those who cannot furnish these evidences often forfeit the right to receive them from others.

The blind theologian John M. Hull, whose memoir we discussed in the last chapter, found that in conversation the sighted regularly misconstrued his silences to mean that he wanted to stop talking when in fact he was simply pondering his response. This was because he did not mark out the peaks and troughs of attention in the usual way by looking at people.[54] At social gatherings, pauses for thought of this sort often resulted in his interlocutor walking off to go and talk to someone else.

The philosopher Havi Carel, who suffers from a rare respiratory condition, has described the effect on strangers of her occasionally needing to wear an oxygen mask:

> I have long given up trying to address, or even process, the looks I get, as well as their hidden, and not so hidden, meanings. I am much less social. I walk in my own groove, oblivious to others' stares, whispers, awkwardness. I have to soldier on, because

we see strangers on the street every day. And the aftershock of internalizing the stares and whispers has to be contained, triaged, suppressed. I feel more alone now because others cannot understand the contours of my world. I no longer walk in their tracks, share their freedom, take for granted the commonality of health, its hegemony, its normalizing force.[55]

In this instance, it is tempting to conjecture that the sight of the mask was sufficient for the whole of Carel's identity to be assimilated into a gestalt of a more alarming disability. Somewhere, the healthy and the able-bodied know that to become ill is to lose agency on a grand scale. Because they are emotionally contagious creatures, they suspect that being around it could result in a loss of *their* agency. If Merleau-Ponty was right that movements in general are ways of enabling intentional states to pass from one human being to another, then it might be in some sense 'natural' to treat deviant bodily deportments as contagious.[56] The most common defence against this fear takes the form of denying peer status to the sick other. That, surely, was the purpose of the stares, whispers and awkwardnesses that others visited on Carel. We are suggesting that their situation invites comparison with that of the infant who would prefer others not to do anything with him.

It is because of the primacy of mirroring in human affairs that the sick are at a disadvantage in most interaction orders. They feel vulnerable in case others write them off pre-emptively as bad reciprocators. They also have reason to believe they are 'not themselves' as a result of the illness. As Robert F. Murphy observed in *The Body Silent* (1987): 'their ways of thinking about themselves and about the persons and objects of the external world have become profoundly transformed. They have experienced a revolution of consciousness.

They have undergone a metamorphosis.'[57] It is not unusual for a person newly diagnosed with a major disease to be so disoriented by the news that they feel disconnected from the world at large. The initial shock of the diagnosis may even result in a temporary impairment of cognitive function.

But humans can choose what to mirror. The healthy and the able-bodied sometimes achieve this realization negatively, when they decide with hindsight that they have mirrored too much and seek to highlight dissimilarity. The writer and psychotherapist Kathlyn Conway found that when she was diagnosed with breast cancer, her friends were initially very supportive.

> As time goes on, people's reactions become more complicated. Once they absorb the news, they begin to protect themselves from their own feelings of vulnerability. Sometimes this means convincing themselves that they are different from me. They reassure themselves that by eating carrots or exercising they will be spared. They ask questions that leave me feeling blamed. Is there breast cancer in my family? Do I eat red meat, or meat treated with antibiotics? Does my diet contain fat? Do I exercise? Have I been under a lot of stress? I begin to feel set apart, isolated, and viewed as responsible for this cancer.[58]

Much worse, of course, is when clinicians – people who are members of a caring profession – refuse even minimal mirroring. People with potentially fatal conditions often complain that their physician fails to acknowledge them as people. They either communicate the brute fact of the diagnosis and invite the patient to come back for more tests or, no less frequently, the diagnosis has the effect of making every other aspect of their humanity irrelevant. Robillard, who lived with motor neurone disease for thirty years, was constantly confronted by his clinicians' inability to see anything other than his diagnosis.

> There is something about having a fatal disease that immediately renders the diagnosee less worthy, and having fewer prospects, than others. The image of the life of the fatally ill leads to comments like the physicians telling me to go home, take Valium, get death counselling, and prepare to die . . . It is a social text, shared by most people in society and reproduced in their remarks. There is an alternative text that says one lives until one dies, but one does not hear it much. When the patient does hear this formulation – that life is not over until it is over – it can sound like it is being introduced as a corrective to the negative view of terminally ill individuals.[59]

Memoirs written by people with serious illnesses often contain passages in which the writer wonders if clinicians will not only treat them sympathetically but vouchsafe them some token of commonality. Tokens of commonality are promises of *sane* mirroring. Often patients look for them without the doctor or the nurse knowing. Conway would scour her doctors' degree certificates hanging on the walls of their consulting rooms to see if they had attended the same universities as her. She was curious about their names. Were they WASPs or from Irish Catholic stock, like her? About her oncologist, the ambiguously named Dr Moore, she has this to say:

> She is a graduate of Smith College and Columbia University medical school, so I assume that she is upper class and Protestant. She must be about fifty. But she is at that point

in middle age when she could look older or younger at any moment. Her glasses make her look grandmotherly, but she treats me as an equal; she strikes me as being someone with whom I could be friends. I imagine she makes everyone feel this way.[60]

Albert Robillard took against agency nurses because:

> they could not locate me in their conversations. The 'me' they could locate with a generic person, but it was not the me that lived in Hawaii, had friends, worked, and had a history in Hawaii and the Pacific Islands. These nurses could talk about where they were from, where they had gone to nursing school, where they had worked, and where I have lived and worked on the u.s. mainland.[61]

With local nurses 'there was a reciprocity of highly detailed knowledge that located both me and them'. When the endocrinologist David Rabin was first diagnosed with motor neurone disease, he was dismayed that the physician who diagnosed him displayed

> no interest in me as a person, and did not make even a perfunctory enquiry about my work. He gave me no guidelines about what I should do, either concretely – in terms of daily activities – or, what was more important, psychologically, to muster the emotional strength to cope with a progressive degenerative disease.[62]

The subtitle of Rabin's *New England Journal of Medicine* article 'Isolation from My Fellow Physicians' makes the point that reciprocity is a vital commodity and, in many respects, the one that turned out to be in shortest supply. These are all examples of awareness by sick and disabled people that others can choose what to mirror in them.

The sociologist and disability activist Irving Kenneth Zola described an experiment he undertook as a participant-observer at Het Dorp, a 65-acre village located in Arnhem in the Netherlands, specifically designed to house four hundred severely disabled adults. Although he was disabled, Zola was mobile, occasionally using crutches. Yet in order to 'gain an awareness of the physical existence of the residents and perhaps some greater ease of communication with them' he decided to spend his time at Het Dorp in a wheelchair.

> As soon as I sat in the wheelchair I was no longer seen as a person who could fend for himself. Although [his friend, Johann Metz] had known me well for nine months, and had never before done anything physical for me without asking, now he took over without permission. Suddenly in his eyes I was no longer able to carry things, reach for objects, or even push myself around. Though I was perfectly capable of doing all these things, I was being wheeled around, and things were being brought to me – all without my asking. Most frightening was my own compliance, my alienation from myself and from the process.[63]

Others ignored Zola in the wheelchair, addressing their comments to Metz instead. When he went to eat in the canteen, he thought he would continue to be a focus of interest as a newcomer and a stranger, but in the wheelchair he observed a marked diminution in others' curiosity about him. He was also disturbed by his own willingness to fall in with this judgement. 'Somehow I lost the right of protest. I had accepted their view of me.' It doesn't seem far-fetched to suggest that the residents of Het Dorp feared that disability might be the only aspect of them Zola wanted to see clearly. It was all that he would mirror in them. His inability to resist their debased image of him was a consequence of his reflecting *their* self-alienation. So long as he was not in a wheelchair, he could reflect back their most able-bodied aspects, but as soon as he sat down in it he lost this most valued ability. He was not reflecting back anything they regarded as positive.

Zola imagined that getting into the wheelchair would erase a distance between his subjects and himself, leaving his own identity undisturbed. The residents did not want Zola to be like them. They wanted him to act as a transformative mirror. They wanted him to do something with what he saw. Edward Tronick would say they saw Zola closing off the possibility of dyadic consciousness with them (because it did not involve him giving them something of his own). Donald Winnicott would say they wanted him to 'hold' them.

In infants, imitation and affect synchrony create the sense of a shared endeavour. This is no less true of adults. Holding begins with stable mirroring. It proceeds from the knowledge that we can choose what to mirror. Stable mirroring is an invitation to reciprocity. Stable mirroring in the case of illness betokens resilience on behalf of the other. It is an earnest of safety.

Adepts of narrative-based medicine understood the importance of stable mirroring, which they often treated under the heading 'empathic witness'.[64] Too often this has been misinterpreted merely as a call for empathy. But most writers in the narrative medicine tradition emphasize witness over empathy with witness implying an acknowledgement of separateness. They are as a rule unflinching about how physically demanding witnessing can be. Rita Charon, perhaps the most influential exponent of the narrative approach to medical practice, has defined her goal as the effort 'to strengthen those cognitive and imaginative abilities that are required for one person to take in and appreciate the representation – and therefore the reality – of another'.[65] This requires the practitioner not only to demonstrate empathy by listening to the patient's perspective, but to 'take in' the patient's physical experience while acknowledging their own simultaneous separateness from and relatedness to it. The shared act of narrating what passes between them is a way of extending both the clinician's and the patient's perspective by making them somewhat continuous with one another. As Charon says, it requires real imagination. With these strictures in mind, we might interpret Zola's decision to spend a week in a wheelchair as an indication of his own willingness to endure temporarily what the residents of Het Dorp had to endure. He was signalling a belief that his imaginative powers were irrelevant to the task of bridging the gap between their experience and his own. It is not surprising that they rebuffed him.

There is no empathic witness without imagination. This is the core of truth in narrative-based medicine. But there is also no empathic witness without a capacity to contain one's own bodily perception of the other's experience (potentially: distress, shock, disgust).[66] This is the deep truth of phenomenology. Nevertheless, if these two pre-requisites concerning imagination and containment are met, the mirroring will tend to increase in sophistication and mutuality and the parties will take pleasure in a degree of interdependence. It is at this point that mirroring turns into holding.

It is interesting to compare Robillard's account of his life with what is known about Stephen Hawking's life. Hawking too had motor neurone disease and like Robillard he lost his power of speech in 1985 after a tracheotomy necessitated by pneumonia. Like Robillard, he had an extended team of researchers, postdoctoral and doctoral students, nurses and others who worked alongside him. One of the most striking findings in Hélène Mialet's remarkable book on Hawking and his team is the extent to which Hawking required collaborators to read his mind and do the things he would have done for himself if he'd been able to.[67] He often issued one-word instructions which those around him learned to puzzle out over time. Although he embodied the myth of free-floating scientific genius, in reality he was embedded in a tight web of people and machines enabling him to work and get on with his life. Here he resembles Robillard closely. But the respect and reverence shown to Hawking are unusual. In the public record at least, there is no trace of the humiliations visited on Robillard: of colleagues crossing the street to avoid saying hello, or imputing idiocy to him on the basis of his appearance; or of being shut out of society. To collaborate with Stephen Hawking was an honour sought by many. It was an experience as far removed from shame as any could be. We suggest that it was easy for Hawking's collaborators to bypass his physical infirmities because they had so much to gain from *his* ability to mirror *them*. Once he bestowed that favour on them, they were able to move to a relationship of holding.

When mirroring turns to holding, the nature of the caring relationship itself changes. Whereas in mirroring, the key reward is acknowledgement of peer status, holding-as-caring begins when the holder and the held open themselves up to each other's psychobiological states. Holding is characterized by transient but regular suspensions of ego boundaries, with the aim of creating something new. In cases of illness this can be frightening and may even require courage. But it can also be extraordinarily satisfying. In a very fine paper, the geriatrician Desmond O'Neill has described how his relationship with his elderly mother was enriched immeasurably during the last two years of her life when she was constrained by dementia, 'chair and bed-bound, in a nursing home'. She had become somewhat withdrawn and her speech was no longer as spontaneous as it once had been. O'Neill would 'sit by her bed with laptop, book, or newspaper'.

> I sought to explore past and future worlds through watching DVDs together related to her interests, including musicals, cooking, travel, and gardening. The greatest surprise was how my relationship with my mother deepened and matured during this time; there developed a sense of an equal partnership. Although I have never doubted that my mother loved me and I her, our family emotions are not worn on sleeves and their outward expression is nearly always elliptical. At the end of an hour together during which she had uttered little, she would nearly always say that she had enjoyed the company or told me to remember that she loved me.[68]

By these means, mother and son were able to 'spend time together in a new framework and relational dynamics in which we were more equal and in partnership than ever before. I looked forward to these times with her – a sentiment which some outsiders might find surprising given public perceptions of thriving and life in nursing homes.'

This phenomenon is not written about enough in the literature on care. Good care involves a quest for equality between the caregiver and the care recipient. We noted in our Introduction Ricoeur's view that care is characterized by 'a search for equality in the midst of inequality'.[69] Winnicott too in his late lecture on 'Cure' observed that when a clinician faces a patient,

> we are reduced to two human beings of equal status. Hierarchies drop away. I may be a doctor, a nurse, a social

worker, a residential houseparent – or, for that matter, I may
be a psychoanalyst or a parson. It makes no difference. What
is significant is the interpersonal relationship in all its rich
and complex human colours.[70]

We also noted how the condition of the patient can become part of
the identity of the carer. Carers sometimes talk about it as if they
had it too but happen to be asymptomatic. It is perhaps the most
arresting instance of something new being created out of intersubjectivity in illness.

Equality enables both parties to discover registers of relationship
that would have unattainable without it. This is the message of
O'Neill and of countless carers of people with life-changing illnesses.

On the specific characteristics of professional healthcare

Some professional medical care is so specialized that the clinician
and the patient don't need to engage with one another at all deeply.
Indeed, in a specialty such as radiology, they don't even need to
meet. Interventions in this category usually occur after a diagnosis
has been given or when one is being sought. The clinician is guided
by her knowledge of pathophysiology and by her proficiency in
carrying out a technical procedure. She may not need to know
anything about the personal side of her patients and she can choose
how much of her own personality to bring in to the consultation. In
Western societies, this arrangement is idealized to the point that it
is assumed to be typical of how medicine in general works. In fact,
it is very unrepresentative of Western medical practice as a whole
and accounts for only a small but important proportion of medical
treatments.

Surveying the consultation from the patient side, we find a conspicuous interest in being known as a person. In 2005 the Mayo Clinic invited 192 patients seen in 14 specialties to give their opinion on what constitutes a good doctor.[71] The patients' responses were then grouped to define seven distinct categories of ideal physician behaviours. The categories were strikingly intersubjective in character.

1 Confident: 'The doctor's confidence gives me confidence.'
2 Empathetic: 'The doctor tries to understand what I am feeling and experiencing, physically and emotionally, and communicates that understanding to me.'
3 Humane: 'The doctor is caring, compassionate, and kind.'
4 Personal: 'The doctor is interested in me more than just as a patient, interacts with me, and remembers me as an individual.'
5 Forthright: 'The doctor tells me what I need to know in plain language and in a forthright manner.'
6 Respectful: 'The doctor takes my input seriously and works with me.'
7 Thorough: 'The doctor is conscientious and persistent.'

We think it likely that if these same patients had been asked to choose between technical competence and intersubjective capacities, they would have come down heavily in favour of technical competence. But it is entirely consistent with the developmental basis of care that patients should foreground these characteristics. It is tempting to conjecture that we are hardwired to look first for something like mirroring and holding. And perhaps that is one of the reasons why so many clinicians who *could* function solely as specialist technicians invest a great deal of themselves in getting to know their patients.[72]

It is often said that physicians treat patients, not diseases. Contrary to the assumptions of many educated lay people, this is not just a piece of piety. Many diseases present insidiously and affect different people in different ways. A symptom which has great salience for one patient may be insignificant to another with the very same condition. The doctor must therefore get to know the disease through the person in all the person's dimensions. It is a very skilled and demanding business, for it requires not only a mastery of biomedicine but an interest in people and an ability to observe one's own states. A huge amount of implicit communication takes place in a diagnostic consultation, some of which may be clinically important. A patient's state of mind can colour the way he presents in the consulting room just as a doctor's state of mind can strongly colour her clinical judgement. These impediments tend to attract responses based on projection.[73]

The neurologist Andrew Lees has recently described his technique in carrying out first diagnostic consultations with new patients.[74] Diagnostic consultations in neurology are especially serious because an adverse outcome is so often life-shattering. Lees tries to concentrate on the patient's *story* as if he were listening to a riveting lecture and, as far as possible, he suspends all frames of reference. He makes a heuristic assumption that everything the patient tells him is true. He never interrupts the patient but will give nods of encouragement if he senses these are needed. Occasionally, if he feels that the patient is overwhelmed by the act of telling their story, he will say something along the lines of 'I think it is incredible how brave you are and how you manage to do so much.' He tries to get the patient to describe their symptoms in their own words, avoiding medical terms. If a patient says he has had a migraine or a fit, Lees asks him to describe what happened in detail. He focuses not just on the patient's words but on how quickly he speaks, the frequency of pauses, the pitch, tone and volume of his voice and his gestures. When the patient has finished talking, Lees asks him if he is aware of any other changes in his body that could be relevant. He then opens a second phase in the consultation in which he asks the patient about his past medical history and about any medicines the patient is taking (including over-the-counter remedies). This occasionally brings to light other chronic conditions not mentioned by the patient, which might be diagnostically significant. If he suspects a hereditary cause, he may ask if parents, siblings or children could come to the next consultation in the hope of examining them or with a view to gaining permission from the patient to talk to other family members in private. In the third phase of the consultation, he invites the patient to talk about anything relating to the symptom that might be worrying him. The purpose of doing so is to draw out the patient's tacit or unconscious knowledge of the problem. Slips of the tongue and casual remarks are often revealing. If Lees suspects that separate but connected symptoms have been telescoped into a single event, he tries to tease them apart. If the patient has been seen by other physicians and is consulting Lees out of desperation, he may ask, 'What do you expect and what do you hope for from the consultation?' Finally, he asks any family members present if they have anything to add to the story. As neurology is a hi-tech specialty, the patient is usually sent for investigations at this point. Lees usually discusses the investigation, explaining what it involves and what it might reveal.

In our terms, the goal of the consultation is one of mirroring. The nods of encouragement and the expressions of admiration of the patient's fortitude serve to emphasize the patient's ascendancy and to clear away obstacles between Lees and his patient. If all goes well, the terms of a possible dyadic consciousness are set. It is important to note that all kinds of diagnostic hypotheses may occur to Lees in this phase, but they are not permitted to eclipse other possibilities. In the second phase, Lees brings his own identity as a doctor into the consultation. Again, all kinds of physical or even psychiatric hypotheses may be entertained in this portion of the interview, but these too must be held in suspense until the patient has had the opportunity to say more. A consequence of this technique is that a patient is enabled to feel heard. We think there is a non-trivial analogy to be made between Lees's technique and Winnicott's account of play. Lees treats the patient's story as a kind of transitional object. The patient is allowed to invest the consultation with meanings that come from himself and by that means to achieve a brief period of verbal mastery over his symptoms. This surely is one of the reasons why Lees tries to suspend *all* frames of reference. It is really only in the next phase – the phase of investigations – that holding in our sense begins, for it is then that he embarks on a clinical journey with the patient, and must contain the patient's fear of, and despair over, what might be revealed. It is also in this phase that doctor and patient can begin to see the significance of their work together, in an act of mutual ratification as far-reaching as any described by the infant researchers. Lees is in no doubt that what is most therapeutic in the consultation is his own persona: 'the most powerful healer I have is myself and not my prescription pad.'[75]

It could be objected that neurology is an outlier specialty: because of the well-known correlation between neurological symptoms and psychiatric syndromes, neurological diagnoses often require a great deal of psychological sifting. From there it might be suggested that neurologists will need to engage with their patients' and their own personhood more closely than other specialties.[76] But Lees's technique is actually very similar to a model that is widely used in general practice. The UK Royal College of General Practitioners advocates 'relationship-based care'; that is, 'care in which the process and outcomes of care are enhanced by a high-quality relationship between doctor and patient . . . characterised by trust, mutual respect and sharing of power between doctor and patient'.[77] If general practitioners could simply slot their patients into diagnostic templates on the basis of pathophysiology, there would be no need to build up relations of trust, mutual respect and power-sharing with them. It is because they cannot proceed on such a basis that these things are necessary.

In our view, there are two main reasons why they cannot do so. The first and most important reason was adumbrated in Chapter One: people consult doctors not because they have a disease but because something that might be a symptom is interfering with their ability to live their lives as they would wish. As the American physician-writer Eric Cassell has observed, 'The trouble may start with a neuromuscular defect, as in amyotrophic lateral sclerosis, but [its] solution lies in the resolution of problems of living in the world.'[78] The same is in fact true of all conditions. For this reason, the doctor needs to understand what matters to the patient. Cassell argues that disease concepts should be used by the general practitioner as part of the unfolding story of the patient, 'not as distinct and exclusive categories in which the object of diagnosis is to find the category into which the patient fits.'[79] The second reason has to do with the nature of disease itself. Diseases do not form a hierarchy from simple to difficult. And because of symptomatic variability and symptomatic overlap (the same symptoms occurring in widely different conditions) they are seldom diagnosed on a first visit. An illness is not an event; it is part of a process. Perhaps this is one reason why so many consultations in general practice – up to 35 per cent by some estimates – are for so-called medically unexplained symptoms, physical symptoms that lack obvious pathological explanations even after appropriate investigations.

The holding that takes place in professional healthcare nevertheless needs to be supported by certain behaviours that enhance its efficacy specifically in relation to the demands of illness. These behaviours we shall group under the name 'compassion'. We should make it clear from the outset that we do not think compassion should be understood in subjective terms as a mode of sympathy or empathy. It is more akin to a stance or a posture: a set of constraints connected with a professional function. A preliminary list of compassionate behaviours would include the following: demonstrating an interest in the patient as a fellow human being; desisting from making moral judgements about him; being honest with him; saying you do not know when you do not know; perhaps most importantly of all, protecting him from unpredictability by exhibiting an evenness of temper or equanimity; and avoiding cruelty.[80] As we shall attempt to show, compassionate behaviours are not separate from mirroring or holding. Rather, they usually arise in order either to create or sustain a clinical holding relationship. The process of getting close to a patient – close enough to understand what might be wrong with him or her – involves subjecting oneself to some strange, sometimes difficult and confusing experiences. Compassionate behaviours enable the clinician to take advantage of those experiences while offering her and her patient a degree of protection from their most detrimental consequences. They address a form of holding that arises between non-intimates who have been thrown together by a disturbance in the life of the patient.

Consider the first compassionate behaviour on our list: demonstrating an interest in the patient as a fellow human being. It is not always as easy as it sounds. In his most extended account of holding in infancy, Winnicott remarked that 'The holding environment . . . has as its main function the reduction to a minimum of impingements to which the infant must react with resultant annihilation of personal being'.[81] It is a good starting point for any reflection on clinical holding to observe that a seriously ill person is always threatened with 'annihilation of personal being'. And this threat of annihilation is something the patient brings into the room with him. When Albert Robillard's physician told him to 'go home, take Valium, get death counselling, and prepare to die', he was saying in effect that he could do nothing about that threat. Insofar as it affected Robillard and not himself, it had nothing to do with him. When David Rabin's neurologist offered no words to help him 'to muster the emotional strength to cope with a progressive degenerative disease' the same limitation was at work: the physician was heavily defended against his patient because he felt helpless in the face of death. It is important to recognize how deeply rooted in us is the instinct to try out other people's psychobiological states. It is something most physicians learn to master but it requires practice.

To care for someone is to form a psychosomatic system with them. This is one of the reasons why it is often all but impossible to care for a sick other without putting oneself in harm's way. It is part of Ricoeur's 'search for equality in the midst of inequality'.

A physician's wish to 'hold' the patient's fear of death may result in an equal and opposite distortion of the threat of mortality: excessive optimism. In 2000 Nicholas Christakis and Elizabeth Lamont published a study of 343 U.S. doctors' predictions of survival times for 504 patients they had referred for hospice care.[82] On average, the doctors overestimated the patients' survival time by more than 500 per cent. As Christakis and Lamont point out, many doctors are aware that they need to show resilience on behalf of their patients, which means being optimistic, sometimes exaggeratedly so. But one of the striking features about this study was that the predictions were made only to the research team, not to the patients. The patients would have suffered no disadvantage had they made a lower estimate.

Studies like those just cited remind us that physicians routinely lend their own well-being to their patients as a matter of course, through precisely the kind of mirroring that Albert Robillard and Havi Carel were routinely denied. It is a crucial intersubjective precursor of care that enables them to reach their patients' experience. It is also one of the reasons why we must say that medical care relies upon the formation of synergistic systems almost as much as infant care does. Healthcare does not merely remedy deficits or impairments.

Compassionate behaviours in general promote the establishment of mutual trust and discourage attitudes that get in its way. Desisting from making moral judgements about the patient is an example of the latter. The injunction to be honest with the patient requires more discretion. We mentioned in the Introduction the discouragement with which Elisabeth Kübler-Ross's attempts to interview terminally ill patients was met. One might expect the situation to have improved since then, and it has, but there is still considerable room for improvement. Two-thirds of the terminally ill cancer patients recruited in a major U.S. government-sponsored study called 'Coping with Cancer' reported having had no discussion with their doctors about their goals for end-of-life care, despite being, on average, just four months from death.[83] This was in 2008. The evidence is that conversations about prognosis *are* taking place in hospital but that they begin only when the patient is very close to death. In his book *Being Mortal*, Atul Gawande describes his treatment of a 34-year-old woman named Sara Monopoli. Sara was nine months pregnant when an advanced tumour was found on one of her lungs.[84] Following the induction of her baby's birth, Sara began a series of treatments aimed at prolonging her life. In the eight months it took her to die, she underwent four rounds of chemotherapy, which made her very ill (one with an experimental drug that had passed only one of the four phases required for full licensing), whole-brain radiation and a bout of pneumonia. Sara knew she was going to die but she and her physicians, along with her family, avoided talking about how long she might have. In his book, *The Way We Die Now* (2016), Seamus O'Mahony, a gastroenterologist based at Cork University Hospital, described how few doctors were willing to have what he calls the Difficult Conversation with patients who are dying. 'It is much easier,' he writes, 'in the middle of a busy clinic, to order another scan than to have the Difficult Conversation.'[85] When Sara Monopoli developed thyroid cancer from her lung cancer, Gawande realized that there was probably nothing further that could be done for her, but rather than saying so, he allowed her to think that he would operate on her lung once more as soon as the thyroid tumour settled down. 'I even raised with her the possibility that an experimental therapy could work against both her cancers, which was sheer fantasy. Discussing a fantasy was easier – less emotional, less explosive, less prone to misunderstanding – than discussing what was happening before my eyes.'[86] There is almost always something more that can be done. And if the doctor doesn't want to do it, patients and their families often will. It is much easier than accepting the overwhelming sadness of the death of a loved one. And sadness is not the only difficult emotion people seek to avoid. O'Mahony works closely with patients with terminal liver disease. More than once, his patients' relatives have threatened to sue him if he didn't arrange a liver transplant, largely because they felt guilty about their dying family member. The pressure on hospital professionals to reassure everyone that death can be postponed indefinitely is often overwhelming.

Kübler-Ross, as we saw, thought that the denial of death stemmed in part from doctors' and nurses' unwillingness to recognize the reality of death as it applied to themselves. Depth-psychological hypotheses of that sort now seldom appear in medical textbooks. These tend to locate the capacity for misunderstanding in the patient alone.[87]

Compassionate clinicians learn to soften the blow of a diagnosis without misleading the patient. Lees gives the example of telling his patient he has progressive memory loss rather than using the word 'dementia'. Suzanne O'Sullivan has written movingly about her slow abandonment of the term 'psychogenic seizures' and its replacement by 'dissociative seizures'.

In his late essay on 'Cure' Winnicott states that a clinician should not hope to gain in a professional relationship emotional satisfactions that ought to be worked out in private life. There are areas of clinical practice where this can be difficult. One of these has been described in arresting detail by Eric Cassell. He notes that the care of the dying often puts the doctor in a situation of great closeness to the patient. He then makes the following assertion:

> The intensely close connection necessary for effective care of the dying is often interpreted as and feels like strong sexual arousal. All perceptions, even of feelings, are given meaning, and meaning is expressed in all dimensions of personhood, including physically. Most people have no experience of such closeness except sexually, so that is how they feel it in the clinical situation. If physicians are not actively taught to deal with this problem, they may end up ducking discussions of their patients' sexual problems and avoiding examinations of sexual organs. Yet I have rarely encountered doctors who were taught about the problem of sex in medical practice.[88]

This problem is less discussed today than was the case in the late twentieth century, for reasons that are unclear to us. Cicely Saunders, the founder of the hospice movement in the UK and herself a physician, is known to have fallen in love 'once or twice' with patients under her care.[89]

Undoubtedly the most demanding compassionate behaviour is the injunction to protect the patient from unpredictability and chaos. This is not something that is taught in medical schools; it is part of the unofficial curriculum of medical training. It arises chiefly when major illness is or could be within striking distance. Many patients with serious illness want their doctors to absorb as much of their worry as can feasibly be managed. The shock of diagnosis, the impact of disease processes on the patient's normal routine, the fear of treatment, the struggle to manage family life as well as relations with the wider world can all be shattering. Obviously, there are limits to what clinicians can do in such situations. But one of the things they can do is make room for these experiences by broaching them sensitively with the patient. This is essentially a mirroring task. If the patient is admitted for hospital care as an inpatient, clinicians should seek to minimize his suffering and create a space in which important relationships can go on existing. Such actions will be in the service of holding, even if the clinician herself is not the immediate provider of it.

Indeed, we might see the attempts to codify medical ethics such as Beauchamp and Childress's four principles of ethical healthcare – beneficence, non-maleficence, respect for autonomy and justice – as projections of the work of compassion, anchored in the duty to mirror and to hold. Recognition of a sick other's personhood seems to be inseparable from recognition that he or she is in some sense *like me*. The autonomy principle secures the fundamental point that healthcare is of the person – not the disease process. The 'harm principle' also implies this, since it refers to harm to the person. Both raise the question 'What would *I* want in his or her situation?' The stage is set for something like mirroring and holding to translate this intuition into action.

In this chapter, we have sought to describe the psychobiological roots of care without equating these with any of the cultural forms care may take. Mirroring and holding will take different forms in different societies but we hypothesize that some version of them exists in them all. The problem of illness becomes part of the problem of life, of living entities in their environment. Our approach is founded on the possibility of understanding the human response to health and illness as turning on similar fundamental mechanisms. As such, it stands in opposition to what is arguably the most influential approach in the medical humanities today, the approach outlined in Annemarie Mol's book *The Logic of Care: Health and the Problem of Patient Choice* (2008).

Mol belongs to that brilliant constellation of science and technology studies scholars applying Bruno Latour's work to the health sphere. Her work takes the form of ethnographies carried out in clinics, so inevitably the lion's share of her attention is focused on overt caring actions. Mol's main aim in that book was to distinguish what we might think of as Hippocratic care from care as a set of commodities. Her vision is attractive in many respects. We admire her robust social-democratic sensibility, her insistence on the primacy of what it is 'appropriate or logical to do in some site or situation, and what is not', and her aliveness to the dangers of marketization.[90] We also commend her defence of technological adjuncts to care.

Mol sees care as a cooperative enterprise, as do we. 'The logic of care', she writes, 'does not start with individuals but with collectives.'[91] The 'collectives to which we belong . . . frame the care we receive, or the care that might be good for us'.[92] It soon becomes apparent that for Mol these collectives comprise not only other individuals but 'professionals, machines, medication, bodies, patients and relevant others', for care is 'embedded in practices, buildings, habits and machines'.[93] Care 'is a matter of attending to the balances inside, and the flows between, a fragile body and its intricate surroundings'.[94]

Nevertheless, it is clear reading her book that she sees a degree of intersubjective attunement between doctor and patient as a *sine qua non* of care: '[patient and doctor] interact, shifting the action around so as to best accommodate the exigencies of the disease with the habits, requirements and possibilities of daily life.'[95] Professional healthcare by physicians – or 'doctoring' as she calls it – 'depends on being knowledgeable, accurate and skilful. But, added to that, it also involves being attentive, inventive, persistent and forgiving.'[96] Attentiveness, inventiveness, pertinacity and forgiveness are the soil in which mutual attunement between the doctor and the patient grows.

It is not clear that Mol sees anything in care that is *intrinsically* disturbing or unstable. For the most part, this is a possibility she avoids. She may be addressing it obliquely in the following sentences: 'care seeks to nourish our bodies; respects the collectivities to which we belong; reacts forgivingly to our failures; and stubbornly strives for improvement, even if things keep on going wrong; though not beyond an (un-)certain limit, for in the end it will let go.'[97] What sort of 'things' might 'keep on going wrong'? Mol doesn't say. The looseness of this formulation probably isn't coincidental. As a Latourean, she rejects the idea of a knowing 'subject' (a clinician, say) interrogating an 'object' (in this case a patient) and she seeks to give due weight to non-social things and processes, hence her emphasis on 'practices, buildings, habits and machines' and on care as a process of trial, error and coordination. We have no objection in principle to the idea that care draws support from machines, buildings, medical equipment and medical knowledge. But can the logic of care, by virtue of the arrangement of its component parts (however these may be specified), really be so straightforward? Does it really have no systemic disorders of its own? On these questions, Mol is, to say the least, opaque.[98]

Pace Mol, we think a key element of the logic of care is a profound confusion of subject and object. Such confusion is not definitive and almost always has to be overcome. But there are powerful forces at work that drive the participants in any caring relationship towards a blurring of ego boundaries. In our view, the logic of care cannot be elucidated without proper engagement with these phenomena. Care is founded on recognition. It is inherently inclusive. In the first instance it aims to overcome deficits in a needy other by supplying whatever is deemed to be missing. But in fact, the act of responsive recognition soon initiates a process of shared meaning-making. This process can be articulated as a narrative of joint action. The existence of such a narrative and its ratification through shared elaboration leads to the kinds of synergies described in infant research. The highly specialized nature of medical care should not blind us to this fact.

Care-seeking is hardwired into us and offers others powerful ways of knowing us (it is hard to know that we are known without it); it therefore draws upon the most fundamental developmental features of human sociality. In her earlier and much longer book, *The Body Multiple: Ontology in Medical Practice* (2002), Mol presents the clinics where she carried out her ethnographic studies as places that *enact* different kinds of vascular disease (including type 1 diabetes).[99] The disease as it is construed by a vascular surgeon is not the same entity as the disease an endocrinologist goes to work on. Indeed, the 'body' as it is enacted in each of those settings is a different thing. Implicitly, we stand possessed of a wondrous but falsely unified world, always in the making, emergent, incomplete and as fragile and mutable as the practices and processes that bring it into being and hold it together. We take the opposite view. The biological motivational systems that actuate human behaviours in relation to care-seeking and caregiving are unified and can be described satisfactorily in evolutionary (Darwinian) terms. It is not only possible but necessary to describe care as a continuum that can be observed in multiple spheres of human social existence.

We have said little in this chapter about disturbances to biological coregulation in relation to illness. This will form an important subject for discussion in our next chapter, which is about the antithesis of care: abandonment.

3

The Pariah Syndrome

Morality seems to conform to the law of optical perspective. It looms
large and thick close to the eye. With the growth of distance, responsibility for the other shrivels, moral dimensions of the object blur,
till both reach the vanishing point and disappear from view.

ZYGMUNT BAUMAN[1]

Others will avoid you. They do not want to deal with mortality,
yours or their own, or what strikes them as worse than death:
frailty, weakness, disability.

ANNE ELIZABETH MOORE[2]

In June 1979, David Rabin, the director of endocrinology at
Vanderbilt University Medical Center in Tennessee, began to
experience stiffness in his legs. A couple of weeks later, he noticed that
his reflexes had become pathologically brisk. Although he tried to tell
himself that he just had 'restless legs', he suspected that he might have
amyotrophic lateral sclerosis (ALS), the disease known colloquially
in the USA as Lou Gehrig's disease, which is called motor neurone
disease in the UK. This diagnosis was confirmed when he travelled
to a prestigious medical centre away from Vanderbilt to consult a
neurologist specializing in ALS. Like so many people diagnosed with
a serious illness, Rabin's first impulse was to conceal his condition
for as long as possible. He wanted to protect his children from the

knowledge that he had a progressive, incurable illness that would rob him of the ability to speak, eat, move and even breathe. He also 'realized intuitively' that if his colleagues discovered he had ALS it could 'destroy [his] professional life at the medical center'. When, in the autumn of that year, he began to walk with a limp, he told his colleagues that he had a slipped disc. Slipped discs did not frighten them. They regaled him with their own back troubles. 'I was still a full member of the fraternity,' he recalled, 'in excellent standing.' But the limp got worse and he had to use a walking stick to get around. It did not take long for his colleagues to work out for themselves that Rabin had a major neurodegenerative disorder. They began to avoid him. 'How often,' he writes, 'as I struggled to open a door, would I see a colleague pretending to look the other way.' The technicians, the secretaries, the cleaning women were not so churlish and opened doors for him readily, 'even if it was only the door to the men's toilet'. On one occasion, he fell over in a little courtyard just outside the Medical Center's emergency room. 'A long-time colleague was walking by. He turned, and our eyes met as I lay sprawled on the ground. He quickly averted his eyes, pretended not to see me, and continued walking.'[3]

About a year after being diagnosed, Rabin was invited to a scientific meeting in the enclave-state of San Marino in the north of Italy.[4] His legs were weak but he still enjoyed the use of his arms and his speech was unimpaired. When he was seated it was impossible to tell that he had an illness. As he thought he might never be able to attend another conference abroad, he and his wife, Pauline, a psychiatrist, decided to accept the invitation. It was a shattering experience. Because of Rabin's disability, the couple were seated early and for convenience's sake they always chose the table nearest the door. As their fellow guests entered the room, they raced to the remotest part of the dining room. 'If eye contact was unavoidable, there would be a hurried "Hello, David" and off the person would go, almost jet propelled.' The conference participants were all staying in the same hotel, taking the same bus to the conference venue, eating their meals in the same dining room and socializing afterwards in the same bar. But people walked past David and Pauline 'with eyes averted or were suddenly mesmerized by the floor'. The Rabins knew there was nothing unusual about their isolation. But they were surprised by how insensitive people were to their social suffering. They devised a name for what they were going through: the pariah syndrome. David recalled his own neglect of an admired young colleague who was struck down with a brain tumour:

> I always thought up a dozen good reasons to avoid visiting him. Finally, I convinced myself that he really wanted to see only his close friends and family. Of course, I was merely rationalizing. We knew and liked each other, and I failed to go and see him because I would be uncomfortable – not he.[5]

In his original article in the *New England Journal of Medicine*, Rabin pondered why physicians in particular might feel especially inhibited in extending support to a medical colleague and his family. Physicians, he observed, see themselves as healers.

> We dispense treatment, counsel and support; and we represent strength. The dichotomy of being both doctor and patient threatens the integrity of the club. To this fraternity of healers, becoming ill is tantamount to treachery. Furthermore, the sick physician makes us uncomfortable. He reminds us of our own vulnerability and mortality, and this

is frightening for those of us who deal with disease every day while arming ourselves with an imagined cloak of immunity against personal illness.[6]

The story the Rabins went on to tell of abandonment by colleagues and friends is a bleak one, perhaps made more so by David's conviction that they were genuinely grieving for him – they just didn't know how to express their grief.

Their daughter Roni, now a medical journalist at the *New York Times*, described her parents' dealings with friends and colleagues in detail in a superb memoir of her father's illness that came out the year he died. 'He knew why he hadn't heard from his colleagues,' she writes; 'they simply didn't know what to say. ALS was a death sentence. Speaking about it would be trespassing onto emotionally volatile ground, sensitive, forbidden and private.'[7] Some told Pauline they needed her help to face her husband in his broken-down state. Many who visited couldn't bring themselves to ask about his illness. Some also feared the sadness surrounding the family. They thought they were there to distract attention from what was going on. There was also a certain amount of squeamishness arising from the fact that a previously handsome man was becoming, in his daughter's words, 'an eyesore'. His appearance now engendered something akin to xenophobia – his daughter's term – in his healthy peers. Some literally couldn't stand the sight of him. A few friends seem to have feared becoming the object of the sick man's envy. They assumed he was wondering why should they be granted the gift of life when he had to suffer and, in all probability, die.

The Rabins were very clear about the scale of the problem: 'any chronic incurable illness', they wrote, 'also induces a social disease. Patients and their families become pariahs, cast off by many in society who are unable to face them. Thus, they contend not only with their illness but also with the response it evokes.' In their case, it took the form of being shunned by 'a rather large group of people' they used to see quite regularly before David's illness. 'We never heard from many of these people again . . . We had been reclassified as pariahs, social outcasts.'[8] Their self-esteem was damaged 'inexorably'. 'We could not escape the feeling that we must in some way be responsible.' Some acquaintances and friends went to extraordinary lengths not to ask about David when they met Pauline or one of their children. Roni Rabin's account of the secondary stigma she experienced as a child is exceptionally powerful:

> People were avoiding us.
>
> It was happening everywhere: in the corridors of the hospital, in Dana and Leora's classrooms, at movie theaters before the lights went out. In the supermarket, at the bakery, in line at the bookstore. People slinking around corners, looking straight ahead to avoid eye contact, pretending to be self-absorbed. It happened after dinner, before Grand Rounds, throughout cocktail parties. In restaurants, at the park, in our own driveway.[9]

When they turned to explore the origins of this unacknowledged 'social disease', the Rabins homed in on social factors. They noted that American society in the late 1970s and early '80s was highly individualistic. The sick were segregated from the well by being confined to hospitals or nursing homes:

> The blind, the deaf, and the handicapped are housed in special enclaves which obviate any need to know how to

relate to these people. We take pains to segregate even those who are at risk for developing illness. Thus we have created retirement centers which offer advantages to the elderly but also serve to isolate them.[10]

Media images celebrated youth and vitality. The Rabins also pointed to a narrowing in the average person's range of life experiences, with fewer and fewer people having any experience of caring for people with chronic conditions, even as these were becoming more prevalent.

Let us say straight away that we find the social-psychological explanations provided by David, Pauline and Roni Rabin very compelling. We need first-hand accounts of how these dynamics play out in real life and the contributions of the Rabin family retain a signal importance in fulfilling that task. There is no doubt that the ill and their close others are marginalized in Western societies, at immense cost, both financially and morally. Scholarship owes the Rabins a great debt of gratitude for drawing attention to the pariah syndrome, which is much more common than many people suppose.

In this chapter, we nevertheless want to explore the pariah syndrome in a more cross-disciplinary way: one that moves beyond social psychology to take account of biology, neuroscience and sociology and that looks at how the body mediates social relationships more generally. The pariah syndrome, as we see it, is merely the most extreme expression of abandonment with which all ill people are threatened. Abandonment, in our conceptual framework, is the opposite of care. It involves refusing to meet the experience of the sick other. As such, it involves denying him or her mirroring, holding and compassion. In the last chapter, we set the social world to one side in order to focus on the intersubjective precursors of care. Of course, in the real world, the context in which care is given has powerful effects on its efficacy. In this chapter, we will include more of the social world, while continuing to pay special attention to the psychobiological aspects of abandonment. This difference of approach reflects the nature of our subject matter: care often takes place *despite* or in defiance of the social context; abandonment almost never does, not least because the social context of WEIRD societies is deliberately organized in such a way that care is driven back into the private sphere. It has become virtually impossible for a lay person to respond meaningfully to someone else's illness in a WEIRD society without putting himself or herself in the role of a close other.

Accordingly, in what follows, we attempt to explain why abandonment is not just a possibility in WEIRD societies, but a strong probability. Our discussion will unfold in three parts. In the first, we will draw attention to the biological strengths that groups of healthy humans can offer one another in the face of adversity. One of the most important of these is the building up of shared autonomic resilience, which enables the individual to harness the physiological power of the group. We will argue that WEIRD societies are set up in such a way that it is harder for the individual to draw upon these strengths. Crucially, this affects those who might support a sick person as much as the person with the illness, and the consequences are often devastating. In the second part, we develop this theme by considering the ways in which healthy individuals help one another to cope with a strangeness that is intrinsic to ordinary embodiment and surveying some of the ways in which illness might obstruct those processes. These help to explain some of the incomprehension that can take root suddenly once illness enters the picture in relationships that were previously stable. Finally, we turn to the related question of the impact of this phase of modernity on how most people think about and indeed live out our notions of health, the body and death.

The social and the biological come together differently in different societies. We will show that there are aspects of bodily experience that our modernity summons up and 'thematizes' and others which it suppresses and renders almost meaningless. Social arrangements don't just harness biological potentials (though, to be sure, that is one of the things they do), but invest them with social meanings that themselves can reinforce or weaken those potentials. A convincing analysis has to get to grips with the traffic moving in both directions: with the power of the biological to channel the force and creativity of the group most effectively, on the one hand, and with the power of the social to magnify or diminish the biological in accordance with its own norms and purposes, on the other.

The biological strength of the group

We begin, then, with a thought experiment. Suppose Rabin had been struck down with ALS before modern neurology existed. Let us picture him, not in Nashville, but in continental Europe some time in the seventeenth century. We will allow him a comparable level of social eminence and easy circumstances. At first, he would have been seen as suffering from a mysterious and incapacitating illness. As his functioning declined, he would probably have spent more time at his home in bed. We would soon be in the territory of what the French historian Philippe Ariès famously characterized as 'tame death'.[11] Tame death was a Catholic death and its key ritual was the deathbed scene: a public display of repentance and acceptance of God's will. It starts off from the assumption that death is something that happens to all of us. It is not particularly frightening. What matters is that the individual accepts the fate of mankind and does so with the support of a community that somehow manages to integrate dying into the flow of life. In most cases, there would be religious consolations of various kinds: readings from scripture, prayers individual and collective, a psalm might be sung, there might even be rituals involving bodily movements (kneeling, standing, bowing, genuflecting and so on). We take it as read that in most of the world's major religions something very similar to tame death obtained for centuries.

Now let us move our protagonist on a century, into the 1700s, when, as a privileged, educated man, Rabin was entitled to be more individualistic. We find him confronting death as a universal predicament and calling forth all the resources of his individuality. We might conjure up a deathbed scene similar to that of the philosopher David Hume. According to Adam Smith, Hume encouraged his friends to talk openly to him about the fact that he was dying: 'so far from being hurt by this frankness, he was rather pleased and flattered by it.'[12] Hume devised speeches in the style of Lucian's *Dialogues of the Dead* in which he asked Charon, as the boatman of the Styx, for more time in which to undertake corrections of his works and to observe with relish the decline of superstitious practices. These were staged at Hume's bedside and his many friends were pressed into service to take part in his unfolding demise until he was too weak to receive them. (Hume did not have a major neurodegenerative disease to contend with; he is thought to have died of abdominal cancer.)

Four aspects of group functioning are worth noticing in both these scenes. First, in both cases, the deathbed scene provided an occasion in which the individual's relation to the group was affirmed. Boswell may have urged Hume to make a deathbed conversion to Christianity but in the end he had to accept the fact that Hume was 'indecently and impolitely positive in incredulity'.[13] Boswell had been coopted against his will into an atheistic but collective celebration of death and dying. Second, by sheer force of numbers, the group supported not only the dying person but its individual members. This is one of the things that distinguishes some contemporary southern European societies from their WEIRD counterparts. When you fall ill in Sicily, one of your biggest problems will be the large number of well-wishers crowding into your living room. You may wonder when you can decently ask them to leave. A very important consequence of approaching illness as a collective problem as the Sicilians do is that it enables the supporters of the sick person to draw strength from one another. The risk of becoming the sick person's supporter of last and only resort is consequently much lower than it would be in WEIRD societies. Third, through the shared ritual of prayers and religious observances in the case of tame death, and by acting out mock classical speeches in Hume's case, the group was bound together by common sets of 'regulating rhythms', a fact of enormous importance, as we shall see. And fourth, the circumstances of death were given meaning by a set of beliefs and values that made death not only acceptable but, from a certain point of view, desirable.

These four characteristics point us towards the foundational importance of the group in managing difficult experience. This is not just a matter of social harmony; it reaches down into the biological. In the last chapter, we described how infants learn to regulate themselves and to coregulate with others rhythmically. They move in and out of sync with their carers and in this way come to manage their homeostatic balance. If they find they are too aroused by the caregiver's gaze, they can turn away and lower their heart rate, settle their breathing and slow the pace at which glucocorticoids enter their blood stream. As infants develop, they become more resilient, where resilience refers to the capacity to move from the stress response to a previously established homeostatic balance. We noted that stress is a double-edged sword. If it's too challenging, the infant's resilience will be impaired, but if it's too weak, he will be unable to take advantage of the predictable climaxes of affect that enable the brain to develop in quite specific ways. Play, we observed, was often most pleasurable when it involved a heightened stress response. But to reach that point, something else was essential: the child had to feel safe. The stress response thus enables system-wide physiological states that facilitate our being in the world: it tells us when we are under some sort of threat, when we are safe and when we can have fun. And rhythm is critical to how it does all of these things. In the case of the baby, the stress response usually begins as a response to multimodal, rhythmically patterned attempts to incorporate her into communal living. These may distress her in part because they are unfamiliar: they do not feel predictable or under her control. But over time, as she learns to weather them and interact with them, they become a source of pleasure.

Rhythm continues to be crucial in adult life because so many of our biological systems use it. Most of us can think of a rhythmic activity we enjoy: it might be something as simple as walking, listening to music or taking part in a sport. A baby in the womb can hear its mother's heart beat at roughly sixty to eighty beats a minute. It 'listens out' for that rhythm when it enters the world. It's why a baby is often easier to soothe when it is held by its mother on the left-hand side, where the sounds of her heart are audible.

This rhythmic seeking behaviour can be seen even in casual interactions between grown-ups. What happens when two strangers meet? Most people would concede that whatever form their interaction takes is likely to be the product of cultural learning: whatever assumptions each brings to the interaction is likely to influence its outcome.

Humans in the face-to-face domain also communicate with one another directly through bodily gesture. This was the territory

Goffman conquered for sociology. Some of this communication is visible through proximity, posture, gestures, facial expressions, the prosodic features of the voice, turn-taking in conversation and a host of other features of ordinary human interactions. All of these bodily signs are profoundly rhythmic and they can all be turned into the stuff of mirroring. We gauge how close the other person wishes to stand and position ourselves accordingly; we determine our posture in response to theirs; we may approximate their gestures and facial expressions, or speak at a similar pitch, intonation and rhythm to them; and we can time our interventions in the conversation in ways that may put them at their ease.

This mirroring conveys information about recognition. Meaning is extracted from it. Consistent with the argument of the last chapter, in the transactions just described both parties will attempt to use one another as mirrors in which they hope to find something of value about themselves reflected in the other's behaviour towards them. We will also be bound to ask whether they see the interaction as fundamentally contractual, based on the realization of reciprocal benefits, or whether it might have the potential to go beyond that to something less conditional. These are considerations that make deep sense in evolutionary terms.

But there is a more recondite domain of *physiological* communication that is no less important in our story. This is the domain of neurobiological coregulation. The face has a special role in this story. According to the neuroanatomist Stephen W. Porges, evolution by natural selection enabled us to convey an unusually wide range of signals to one another through our faces.[14] Signals conveying safety were paramount. We scan the faces of others to determine whether it is safe to be in their presence; others do the same to us. Much of this appraisal-work takes place out of awareness and at astonishing speeds. The face is a reliable guide to the state of the viscera because the muscles that govern facial expression are controlled in the same portion of the brainstem that regulates heart rate and breathing, by way of the vagus nerve. If we feel unsafe, our heart rate increases, our breathing becomes heavier and our blood pressure rises. These responses are initiated by the autonomic nervous system and do not need to pass through the thinking part of the brain. They trigger the physiologically costly fight–flight response associated with the sympathetic nervous system. If we feel safe, on the other hand, our heart rate decreases, our blood pressure falls and our breathing reverts to its normal rate. These visceral markers confer a further rhythmical dimension on the interaction. For Porges, this gives the face and the head a lot of work to do. If we want another person to feel safe in our company, we need to register that we feel safe in theirs. We need to allow a great deal of expression to show in our faces, we should not be afraid to meet their gaze, we should gesture with our heads and speak without fear. Porges calls this set of responses the social engagement system or SES. The SES operates dialogically with other people's SESs. The theory of the SES suggests that intersubjectivity is built on shared bodily experience. It is rhythmical through and through. If the mutual attunement of mother and baby is of the same order of complexity as the choreographing of a ballet, the same is true of adult interactions. But it is largely hidden from view because of the centrality of language in adult communications. The point about the SES is that not only does it provide a constant source of feedback about the quality of the communication taking place between two people, but it enables both parties to regulate their own and each other's autonomic arousal levels. This interpersonal neurobiological regulation of autonomic states is something we depend on, in ordinary life, most days. It is shared life in action.

If we loop back to Rabin's experience in the late twentieth century, we are confronted with the absence of a group in which messages of safety can circulate. A few intrepid individuals made it their business to befriend Rabin and his family, but they were exceptions. No group affirmed him as a member. Neither was there much support for his supporters. He repeatedly experienced 'the failure of acquaintances and friends to even inquire about me when they met my wife and children' and his children felt they had 'a distinguishing mark, a sign on [their] forehead: dying father'.[15] There was, moreover, no means of rhythmic coregulation. Rabin's condition meant he could no longer convey his intentions, interests and feelings by moving his body with confidence. In Trevarthen's terms, the possibility of intersubjective motor control with others was lost. The revulsion that overwhelmed so many of his acquaintances as his disease progressed may have been in part a response to this loss: without the expected visible means of rhythmic coordination, friends and acquaintances didn't know how to be with him any more.[16] But above all, there was no shared meaning-making, only the anomie of certain death. David had been raised as an Orthodox Jew and enlisted the services of a rabbi towards the end of his life. Yet religion could not fulfil the function it had served for thousands of years, that of including the individual in communal life at its most exalted and mundane. Let us not be misunderstood. We are not proposing that WEIRD societies should embrace religion again. We do, however, think that religious groups have managed to invest sickness and death with collective meanings that enable them to face both in a steadier and more altruistic way than post-religious societies.

Members of the Rabin family observed repeatedly that others wanted to help them but felt powerless to act on that wish. Humans are emotionally contagious creatures. We do not need language to pick up one another's moods. When help is needed, we know it, most of the time. Over the last two decades, academic psychologists have argued persuasively that the desire to alleviate the suffering of others is a powerful human instinct.[17] There can be no doubt that some degree of automatic sympathy would be highly adaptive. Darwin himself in *The Descent of Man* (1871) said that 'those communities, which included the greatest number of the most sympathetic members, would flourish best, and rear the greatest number of offspring.'[18] Recent work by researchers at Stephen W. Cole's lab has even suggested that compassion is good for health and longevity.[19] But the fact that it is in some sense 'natural' does not make it easy or automatic. A decisive factor – we suggest, the most important one – is the attitude of the larger group. Individuals always feel stronger in relation to adversity as part of a group in which messages of safety circulate regularly and repeatedly. These enable the group to coregulate and in the process gradually to build up its own resilience in relation to the challenges it faces – a process that is sometimes called 'weathering together'.[20] It is weathering together that is so compromised in WEIRD societies. For most of our evolutionary past, humans typically lived in groups of anywhere between 25 and 50 people and seldom more than a hundred.[21] These people were bound to one another largely though not exclusively through ties of kinship. In that situation, the protective function of the group was very often the difference between life and death. The primary function of group life is the provision of safety. This fact remains deeply anchored in human biology. Even if it is played out in scenes that seem remote from the struggle for existence our ancestors had to endure, it continues to be the most important biological principle mediating human social interactions today.

Individuals acting alone or almost alone can be very creative and immensely useful to people in need, but it is harder to stay the course as an individual. This fact surely accounts for the well-known phenomenon whereby the immediate response to an announcement of illness is one of concern and sympathy, but trails off sharply after a few weeks. In WEIRD societies a sick person's many well-wishers will often be unknown to one another; they do not constitute a group in our sense because their actions are not coordinated. How very different from the arrangements instituted by Barbara Rosenblum and her friends described in Chapter One. What Rosenblum demonstrated was that the adversity attendant upon major illness can be significantly blunted by a group that agrees to constitute itself as a group.

In conclusion, there is a threshold of neurobiological synchrony that fosters group resilience in the face of all kinds of adversity, including illness and bereavement, and the way to reach that threshold is through: a) public expressions of group affiliatedness; b) the promise that supporters of the sick person will themselves be supported; c) rituals and other activities fostering shared bodily rhythms; and d) a willingness to interpret what happens in a culturally meaningful way that is in some sense profound and, in optimal circumstances, ecstatic. What happens in our modernity is that the social context deprives us of these props. WEIRD social arrangements largely ignore the potentials of neurobiological synchrony.

Irreducible bodily strangeness

Writers in the critical phenomenological tradition tell us that there is something intrinsically disturbing about *healthy* bodily experience that cannot be fully disguised culturally.[22] We require others to ratify our experience for us, usually by offering us an acceptable version of ourselves through *their* embodiment. More than half a century ago, Frantz Fanon found that when he entered a train carriage, other passengers moved away so as not to have to sit beside him. They held him accountable to their own racial stereotype of the Black man, regardless of how he actually behaved. It's still a common experience for Black people in predominantly White societies. People with disabilities report similar experiences. And of course, feminist critical phenomenologists have drawn attention to the ways in which girls and women are robbed of the feeling that their experience can be normative. Iris Marion Young in her classic essay 'Throwing Like a Girl' notes that if you are brought up to doubt your bodily capacities you will be timid. The world your body reaches out to will be denuded of possibilities. You will, moreover, be at a disadvantage relative to those who are raised to be confident in their bodily capacities.

> The young girl acquires many subtle habits of feminine body comportment – walking like a girl, tilting her head like a girl, standing and sitting like a girl, gesturing like a girl, and so on. The girl learns actively to hamper her movements. She is told that she must be careful not to get hurt, not to get dirty, not to tear her clothes, that the things she desires to do are dangerous for her. Thus she develops a bodily timidity which increases with age. In assuming herself as a girl, she takes herself up as fragile.[23]

Young concludes that 'the general lack of confidence that [women] frequently have about our cognitive or leadership abilities, is traceable in part to an original doubt in our body's capacity.'

What this tells us is that even normative healthy (and perhaps implicitly White, male, able-bodied) experience depends on others to help ratify and renew it more or less constantly. If, as feminist writers often say, 'autonomy takes two', so does bodily well-being. Healthy adults are typically subject to an unsettling aspect of embodiment which they suppress by recruiting others to dampen it down for them (which is to say that they deploy intersubjectivity against it). The most common way of doing this is to look for people who are *like them*.

This obviously puts the sick at a disadvantage. In this section, we will consider three aspects of what we have termed ordinary embodied strangeness. Taken together, they enable us to describe a gradient of bodily interdependence ranging from a fairly subtle interaction that typically enables us to repress our bodily experience in the moment in order to take advantage of opportunities and possibilities in the environment (a contractual commitment, in the terms of Chapter One), through to a historically sedimented sense of what it's like to be with another person, to a more physiologically intense interaction based on enhancing one another's sense of safety (an embedded commitment).

Waldenfels and allopathos

Growing up involves learning to cope with a wide range of bodily discomforts. Such discomforts are part of what we might call psycho-somatic normality. Adapting to the rhythms of one's psychosomatic reality is a productive process that enables the self to develop, not just the body. According to the German phenomenological philosopher Bernhard Waldenfels, there is nevertheless something irreducibly uncanny about bodily experience that we need others' help to transform.

Consider this hypothetical situation. I am asleep and wake up to hear the front door of my house open at 3 a.m. I don't just hear the sound of the key turning in the lock or the movement of the door;

I hear my son coming home after a night out. I wonder why he's so late. Is he all right? Should I get up and check? There is a time-lag between the sounds made by his entrance and the thoughts and feelings these magnetize. Waldenfels calls this magnetization 'the birth of sense out of pathos', where pathos is defined etymologically to mean 'undergoing or suffering [an experience]'.[24] The time lag is a liminal space in my experience. It separates me from my body but is also somehow still 'in me' in the form of sensory memories. According to Waldenfels, we manage this alienness by allowing bodily experiences to collect meanings. This is a highly creative process, for my bodily experiences are both about me and not about me. I do something to them that pitches them into a 'beyond' where they become at once more meaningful and less meaningful: more meaningful because they have been absorbed into a rich human context, and less meaningful because they live on only as husks denuded of the strangeness with which they originally struck me.

There is, of course, nothing original in the claim that one of the blessings of health is that it allows us to repress our bodily experience to better take advantage of opportunities and possibilities in the environment. It goes back at least as far as Charles Sherrington's *The Integrative Action of the Nervous System* (1906).[25] The value of Waldenfels's contribution is that it describes this process of repression in detailed experiential terms. In effect, he sees it as having a twofold character, positive and negative. The positive side invites comparison with Winnicott's definition of transitional experience, for Waldenfels is saying that the repression of the body allows me to connect and separate inner and outer reality in my own way. It is a process over which I can exercise a measure of discretion, which is the source of its 'transitional' character (in the Winnicottian sense). In the example just given, I *could* have felt relief that my son had come home but I chose to make him an object of concern. The negative side exists as a penumbra shadowing the positive side in the knowledge that physical experience qua physical experience can never be fully integrated. It is always ineluctably alien and in important respects outside our control.

My encounters with others reinforce my sense that the corporeal is profoundly alien. When I see another person for the first time my responsiveness is aroused: I do not know his intentions. 'The other's otherness,' Waldenfels writes, 'which overcomes and surprises us, disturbs our intentions before being understood in this or that sense.'[26] The discomfort we feel is visceral. And yet, at the same time, I am impelled to give him ontological recognition as a person, that is, as someone who is *like* me. He is both other and not quite other. When he looks at me, I do not know what to expect. This is analogous to the moment I hear the door open in the hypothetical situation described earlier on, for in both cases there is a huge drive to integrate the strangeness of the moment into something familiar. Moreover, I am alien to him. He is looking at me as someone who is like him and yet not him. I glimpse myself being seen as another. I hear someone calling my name and I hear myself referred to as another. The marks others use to relate to me do not all belong to my 'sphere of ownness'. I become estranged from myself – I have an experience of what Waldenfels calls *Ichfremdheit* (ego or self-alienness). I realize that I carry an abundance of otherness in me, by virtue of the language I speak, the upbringing I received, the culture I live in and so on. Waldenfels puts it this way: 'my own body is a half alien body, charged and even over-charged by intentions, but also desires, projections, habits, affections and violations, coming from others.'[27] Specific others merely particularize this more general experience of otherness. Waldenfels says that the birth of meaning out of pathos leads back to a sort of *allopathos* – a condition of affecting and being affected by others. Others disturb me and at the same time shape my being. Because of them, I can never settle into my own body as something exclusively mine. This drives me to seek out relations of trust with others and to struggle to engage with them.

Waldenfels stands on the shoulders of Merleau-Ponty, who describes how we find ourselves in an intercorporeally constituted intersubjective world. Waldenfels seems to us to amplify what is most valuable in Levinas's philosophy: the idea contained in Levinas's late work *Otherwise than Being* (1974) that in allowing ourselves to be stirred by the presence of another person, we discover our own vulnerability.[28] The other, for Waldenfels, is not, as early Levinas would have had it, 'absolutely transcendent' but immanent within us in the form of a shared experience of vulnerability. And we encounter that vulnerability through the body as much as through cognition.

The Boston Change Process Study Group and 'implicit relational knowing'

In 1994 a group of developmental psychologists based in Boston, Massachusetts, with an interest in psychoanalysis came together to consider what light, if any, infant research might shed on the process of therapeutic change in adults. Some of the most important figures in infant research who also happened to be psychoanalysts, such as Daniel Stern, Ed Tronick and Louis Sander, belonged to this group. The Boston Change Process Study Group, as it called itself, identified deep similarities between caregiver–infant dyads and therapists and patients. The model has proved enormously influential outside psychoanalysis (possibly because it uses almost no psychoanalytic theory).[29] We want to rehearse it here because we think it offers a model of being together with another person that physical illness is likely to challenge. Like Waldenfels, the Boston Group are concerned with the use of the other to create a sense of bodily normality. But where his focus was on the difficulty of arriving at such a sense, theirs is on one of the outcomes of having done so.

The keystone of the Boston Group's model is the concept of 'implicit relational knowing'. Implicit relational knowing is, according to Karlen Lyons-Ruth, 'the domain of knowing how to do things with others'.[30] It is based on long and repeated experience. The predictable climaxes of affect that we create for babies by changing the prosodic features of our voice and face continue to form the armature around which adult communications are woven. But we do not mark them out in quite the same way. Long acquaintance and perhaps even intimacy with a friend means we will know how to be with him or her: what forms of approach will be easy. Some aspects of implicit relational knowing will be conscious. For example, we might share a hobby or an interest with our friend and talk about it a great deal. But the bedrock of implicit relational knowing is the sedimented and internalized *physical* experience of having formed a reliable and familiar affective communication system with them. This gives us a procedural, implicit, nonconscious memory of how to be with that person. The existence of this physical memory is why implicit relational knowing overlaps with, but exceeds, autobiographical memory. We could think of the Boston Group as describing the normal consequences (in health) of Waldenfels's *allopathos*. You end up with a physical feeling of what it's like to be with your good friend X. In the terms of Chapter One, we tend only to have implicit relational knowing with close others or those who are on the threshold of being close.

The theory of implicit relational knowing may shed light on a side of human relatedness that doesn't figure in the language we use to talk about relationships. Lyons-Ruth tells us that implicit relational knowing arises from 'intimate interactions [that] are not language-based and are not routinely translated into semantic form'. We experience implicit relational knowing as a vital *background* experience.

Roni Rabin describes a couple who had long been her parents' closest friends. They would bound into the Rabin home, describe their successful lives and behave as if nothing at all had happened to David. This pretence must have been as stressful for them as it was for the Rabins, but it was all they could manage. Perhaps they should be given credit for their attachment to the old implicit relational knowing they once enjoyed with their friends. Kathlyn Conway recalls that shortly after she was given the all-clear for a breast cancer recurrence, she met a friend for lunch and began talking to her about how traumatizing it was to be treated for cancer. Her friend stopped her immediately and told her they couldn't discuss cancer any more. We might wonder if the friend's reluctance was due in part to the attritional effect of the illness on their pre-existing implicit relationship. Censoring Conway in this way might thus have been a constructive, reparative act. In this area, there is so much scope for misunderstanding.

Porges's Polyvagal Theory and the management of unease

One of the most intriguing implications of Stephen W. Porges's Polyvagal Theory is the notion that compassion is possible only among mammals. Compassion requires us to turn off our defences, most specifically the defences associated with the sympathetic nervous system (the fight–flight response). Porges thinks this is something we are primed to do only with long-trusted others. The Polyvagal Theory thus enables us to see that the activation of the sympathetic nervous system is one of the most powerful factors preventing us moving from a contract-based transactional interaction to a more embedded relationship. It also suggests that with anyone who is not an intimate other, the sense of safety is something that has to be renewed constantly – echoing one of Goffman's core claims about the interaction order. This is much harder when one or more parties to the interaction is stressed. This has been shown in relation to mental illnesses. The Polyvagal Theory has been used to study neurological and physiological mechanisms of borderline personality disorder, depression and extreme dissociative states.[31] In each of these conditions, patients have been shown to have a less forceful vagal brake, more sympathetic activity and more freezing behaviours.

In the wake of the diagnosis of a major physical illness, it is possible for the healthy and the able-bodied to become demotivated to maintain the relationship in the absence of a mutually ratified experience of safety. This was surely one of the factors behind the hesitation shown by so many of the Rabins' acquaintances. And phenomena of this kind often lead the sick person to withdraw. They feel themselves to be a source of depression in others.

Where the Polyvagal Theory really wins is in explaining why those who go to the aid of someone in need often feel better than those who hang back. Helping others directly usually involves using the SES. This in itself is health-promoting because it inhibits both the stress response and physiologically costly freezing behaviours. It might also explain a finding reported by Graham Thornicroft and his colleagues that the most effective interventions for mitigating the stigma of mental illness involved social engagement with those who deemed themselves to be mentally well.[32]

The three capacities we have described in this section – *allopathos*, implicit relational knowing and the neurobiological pursuit of safety – are general human capacities. In the real world, they are channelled by social norms. Here it may be helpful to bear in mind what sociologists call 'habitus'. This is the name given to the particular forms of civilization that individuals take on in order to signal that they belong to the same group. According to Pierre Bourdieu, the chief way in which they do this is via the body.[33] By presenting ourselves in a certain way, we show we know how to inhabit certain kinds of social spaces with others; this in turn means we can command a measure of identification from our peers. The body Bourdieu describes is much more than a placeholder for social markers. Rather, it enables us to indicate a range of expectations concerning the social structure as a whole and to define ourselves as actors in relation to that structure. Bourdieu believed that all habituses are founded on forms of solidarity. The connection between solidarity and safety hardly needs to be stressed. A theory of habitus or something like it is necessary if we are to understand how *allopathos*, implicit relational knowing and the neurobiological pursuit of safety unfold in specific contexts.

The extent to which we consciously attend to *allopathos*, implicit relational knowing and the neurobiological pursuit of safety will be socially determined. The vulnerability that Waldenfels and Levinas regard as a fundamental part of our experience is largely played down today. We seek experiences that minimize it and avoid those that bring it to our notice. Implicit relational knowing is something verbal people especially might want to consign to the background of experience. But the neurobiological pursuit of safety is so all-pervasive that it is virtually impossible not to underestimate it. Again, WEIRD societies largely take *visceral* safety for granted. This was not always the case.

The pariah syndrome and contemporary modernity

It is against this background that the cultural context of illness needs to be assessed. In one of his last, posthumously published books, *The Society of Individuals* (1991), the German sociologist Norbert Elias proposed that sociology might be seen as the study of how community life shapes the motivations of the individual.[34] Elias pointed out that when we talk about individuals nowadays, we assume that such persons are or ought to be autonomous. This is a relatively recent development; Elias dated it to the early seventeenth century. Although we evolved as a species to live in groups, modernity has been characterized by the distinction between what is done individually and what is done collectively and this in turn gave rise to what Elias termed a balance between I-Identity and We-Identity, or the 'We-I Balance'. For most of our history as a species, the We-I Balance was tilted decisively towards the We end of the scale. We lived collectively because it was too dangerous to live individually. The triumph of modern individuality is that it has enabled us to try out new kinds of We-I Balance. Elias pointed out that the We-end of the scale had been transformed every bit as decisively as the I-end. In particular, the most powerful mode of social organization today is the state, a collectivity comprising in some cases billions of people and seldom fewer than millions. Today there are 193 states registered at the UN and many of them participate in transnational supra-state organizations such as the EU, the UN, the WHO, the International Criminal Court and many others. The more developed a state is from an economic point of view, the looser, on average, will be the ties that bind the individual not only to the extended family but to the nuclear family. As Elias puts it, the modern 'state apparatus . . . embeds the individual in a network of rules which is by and large the same for all citizens' and by this means enables a process of mass individualization.[35] Mass individualization is not quite a contradiction in terms. (Arguably, the theory of habitus that Elias played no small part in developing in the 1930s is an attempt to explain it.) Of course, it is not the case that the state is the only meaningful source of group identity. Other institutions such as the family, the school, the world of work and religious and political organizations also play a decisive role in shaping individual mentalities. But in Europe at least, when it comes to illness, the state is overridingly important, as European healthcare systems are supervised more or less directly by the state, which is seen as the supporter of first and last resort in cases of illness. No one who lived in the UK during the SARS-COV2 pandemic of 2019–22 can fail to have been struck by the prime minister's exhortations to the public to get vaccinated to protect themselves 'and our NHS'. For Elias, the truly decisive change, visible from the 1960s onwards, occurred when the family ceased to be inescapable as the primary We-group. 'Many family relationships,' he writes, 'which earlier were obligatory, lifelong, external constraints for many people, now increasingly have the character of a voluntary, revocable union which places higher demands on the capacity for self-regulation of the people concerned, and equally for both sexes.'[36]

In fact, despite a plethora of names applied to our current moment – the era of 'instrumental rationality' (Habermas), post-modernity (Lyotard), liquid modernity (Bauman), reflexive or second modernity (Beck), neoliberalism (Harvey, Sennett) – a remarkable consensus holds among sociologists concerning its core features.[37] One stands out in particular: the 'We' reference points are hollowed out, throwing the subject back on his own resources, leaving him to negotiate with others for recognition with whatever leverage he has at his disposal.

The fact that there are almost as many women as men in paid employment in most WEIRD societies has transformed the balance of economic power between the sexes (for the better!). It has probably been an indispensable precondition for the rise of the modern care industry. At the same time, long-term jobs have become a thing of the past for much of the workforce. Many people's working lives take the form of a sequence of unrelated jobs, in which they never get to build up skills. Fear of losing employment and income is a constant worry. As the American sociologist Richard Sennett has pointed out, we do not value manual labour or the skills that go with it; we value the exceptional and reward it disproportionately.

For the winners in the world of work, the individual is free to move from job to job without incurring any of the penalties imposed on the majority. The net effect has been well described by Ulrich Beck in his book *Risk Society: Towards a New Modernity* (1992):

> the tendency is towards the emergence of individualized forms and conditions of existence, which compel people – for the sake of their own material survival – to make themselves the centre of their own planning and conduct of life. In fact, one has to choose and change one's social identity as well as take the risks of doing so.[38]

The ideal of WEIRD societies is of an individual who is completely self-sufficient: teeming with agency and yet infinitely malleable as circumstances require.

Pierre Bourdieu has lamented the 'shrivelling' of what he terms 'organizing associations' such as churches, trades unions and political parties, which 'guaranteed a sort of "continual enfolding" of a whole world (especially through the organization of sporting, cultural and social activities), thereby giving a meaning . . . to life in general.'[39] In the not-too-distant past these organizing associations had a significant buffering effect against social exclusion, one of the main scourges of the current phase of modernity.

Many of the other main 'We' reference points have become what Beck calls 'zombie institutions' – institutions that are dead but somehow still alive. In an interview, Beck offered the following off-the-cuff characterization of one such institution, namely the family:

> Ask yourself what actually is a family nowadays? What does it mean? Of course there are children: my children, our children. But even parenthood, the core of family life, is beginning to disintegrate under conditions of divorce. Grandmothers and grandfathers get included and excluded without any means of participating in the decisions of their sons and daughters. From the point of view of their grandchildren the meaning of grandparents has to be determined by individual decisions and choices.[40]

Beck is far from idealizing the status quo ante but he is surely right that the obligations that once held the family together as a social unit have become objects of negotiation. Family roles are the outcome of sometimes bitter bargaining where having a place in the family is something that can be taken away, with only feeble rights of redress available to those who lose out.

The combined effect of these changes is that what the sociologist Helen Fein memorably called the 'universe of obligation' – 'the circle of individuals and groups toward whom obligations are owed, to whom rules apply, and whose injuries call for amends' – has for most people in WEIRD societies become smaller and more plastic.[41]

This, as much as anything else, explains why the social networks of the ill become so much thinner. One might expect that in such a situation, the claims of the sick would stand out as especially pressing; but precisely because we invest so much of our dignity in the ideal of autonomy, it is hard to recognize illness as such. Illness becomes, so to speak, a 'reading out of parameter', or, in Goffman's terms, an egregious 'situational impropriety'. We pretend it isn't there, like Rabin's colleague who stepped over him when he fell. Only those who see themselves as a close other will look at it steadily and see it for what it is.

Beck made an important observation when he said that while our modernity doesn't recognize obligations and is somewhat flexible as to values, it is nevertheless very moral-minded. Here, perhaps, we might think of the acquaintances who were 'genuinely grieving' for David Rabin but who stayed away. In Elias's terms, it could be suggested that members of WEIRD societies remain highly attached to the idea of the We-group, but don't trust it very much because they don't trust others to uphold it. They thus find themselves in a classic prisoner's dilemma situation.

There are, in our view, three further specific features of contemporary modernity that complicate relations between the healthy and the ill in ways that have few historical precedents. These show up in assumptions commonly made in WEIRD societies about health, the body and death. They combine to make illness more of an anomaly than it need be. The ill find that they are at grave risk of becoming non-persons.

Consider first the common observation that health is the secular counterpart to salvation. It seems safe to say that health has generally always been seen as desirable. But today, health as an ideal has taken on fresh significance. In the era of tame death, it didn't matter if you died at ten or eighty. From a strict Christian point of view, our time on earth was a probationary period in which we proved our worthiness to enter the kingdom of heaven. Today, if belief in the afterlife hasn't completely died out in WEIRD societies, it has become more nebulous, often taking New Age forms. Health matters because without it we cannot prove our effectiveness as agents in the world. If you become unhealthy you're less likely to hold down a job, find a partner or enjoy any of the security that those advantages typically bring. When Albert Robillard received his diagnosis, a gastroenterologist told him: 'You are lucky your wife did not leave you. Most people in your condition have had their wives split long ago.'[42] The gastroenterologist was not exactly wrong. The risk of divorce appears to be higher when it is the wife who falls ill.[43] As Beck and Elisabeth Beck-Gernsheim point out, the duty to maintain one's health has become a fundamental responsibility in an individualized society.[44] We must look after our health or face the consequences. The individual should eschew behaviours harmful to his health and embrace those beneficial to it. He should eat well, take exercise, and refrain from smoking and from drinking alcohol. If he wants to stave off dementia, he should engage in hobbies that train his brain to accomplish new tasks: he can take up a musical instrument, for example, or learn a new language. Here it has to be said that the consequences of becoming ill are often devastating. People give up jobs and become poorer, more socially isolated and less able to pursue relationships with people on the same footing as before. The financial devastation that often goes with being ill is something which David Rabin does not talk about. Today in the USA, although the number and proportion of medically caused bankruptcies is disputed, it is accepted by virtually everyone that having a hospital admission increases the likelihood of bankruptcy.[45]

Underpinning our notions about health is a more counterintuitive and entrenched set of notions about the body. The Rabins noted that their contemporaries sought to make themselves as invulnerable as possible to bodily experience. Their contemporaries avoided taking public transport and drove a car instead. They sunbathed in the rear gardens of their homes where no one could see them. They sought to live in homes surrounded by high walls. The Rabins interpreted these behaviours as evidence of individualism, but they are much more than that. They constitute an attempt to secure invincibility and control in a world that is no longer constructed on a human scale.

In his book *Flesh and Stone: The Body and the City in Western Civilization* (1994), Richard Sennett suggests that since the late nineteenth century, Westerners have created a world in which many people's bodily experience involved small gradations of effort and was less subject to intrusion than anything our ancestors could contrive. Consider by way of example how we move through space. Trains and cars have revolutionized travel. Unparalleled velocity has 'made it hard to focus on the passing scene'.[46] Driving a horse-drawn coach was a physically strenuous task, especially compared with the physical demands of driving a power-assisted modern car. To navigate a modern city requires a tiny fraction of the physical effort required in previous eras; our era is characterized by the surely unprecedented assumption that there neither is nor should be any need for such effort. 'The traveller, like the television viewer, experiences the world in narcotic terms; the body moves passively, desensitized in space, to destinations set in a fragmented and discontinuous urban geography.'[47] Velocity, speed and escape are crucial dimensions of our relation to cities. Sennett draws a sharp contrast between our era's attitude to the body and that of the ancient world. The major public buildings of fifth-century Athens lay open to the world just as its male citizens went about naked. 'To the ancient Athenian,' Sennett writes, 'displaying oneself affirmed one's dignity as a citizen. Athenian democracy placed great emphasis on its citizens exposing their thoughts to others, just as men exposed their bodies.'[48] Women were clothed and were usually hidden away in enclosed buildings. The citizen in the *agora* expected to be jostled by others no less curious to witness its excitements. The debaters in the assembly or *pnyx* were made vulnerable to the rhetorical stimulation of words. This, Sennett observes, was a polity in which people did not 'think of social instability and personal insufficiency as pure negatives.'[49] People knew that civic compassion 'issues from . . . physical awareness of lack in ourselves'. Here we have a powerful example of how biological potentials come to be invested with social meanings.

Yet it is in relation to death that our helplessness reaches its apogee. Death is the Other of modern life. In a way, it has been for well over a century. Today this alterity takes a different form. Robert Fulton noted as early as 1965 that,

> We are beginning to react to death as we would to a communicable disease . . . death is coming to be seen as the consequence of personal neglect or untoward accident. As in the manner of many contagious diseases those who are caught in the throes of death are isolated from their fellow human beings.[50]

The drive to confine the ill in institutions dates from that period and it is still very much a part of our illness culture. The denial of death among intimates has been with us a long time. Tolstoy portrayed it beautifully in a celebrated passage in his novella *The Death of Ivan Ilyich*:

Ivan Ilyich's chief torment was the lie – the lie that was for some reason acknowledged by all – that he was only ill, and was not dying, and that he only needed to keep calm and undergo treatment, and then something very good would come of it. Yet he knew that whatever they did, nothing would come of it, except for even more torturous suffering and death. And he was tormented by the lie, tormented by the fact that they did not want to admit what everyone knew, and what he knew, but wanted to lie . . . and they wanted him, forced him to take part in this lie himself.[51]

What seems to have intensified steadily in the last quarter of the twentieth century is squeamishness in the face of death. So many people with only *potentially* fatal conditions report that others withdraw immediately.

Many previous writers have observed that the struggle against death is implicitly a collective one and that it always has been. It is hard for members of WEIRD societies to see this dimension of the human relationship to death. Freud observed that there is a tacit social arrangement to behave as if death were not a part of life. In normal times, and under civilized circumstances, we give one another (in Zygmunt Bauman's phrase) permission not to look at mortality, our own or anyone else's.[52] In normal times, the dying or possibly dying individual is felt to wrench that permission away from us unceremoniously. We do not always resent him or her for doing so. In his essay 'Thoughts for the Times on War and Death' (1915) Freud observed that there was no shame in being a soldier about to go off to fight in a war on which the future of the country depends. The social sanction of disbelief, the permission not to look, is withdrawn in such circumstances, out of concern for the person and the group. But generally speaking, we need the permission of others not to look at mortality.[53] Since at least the Romantic period many Europeans have idealized the possibility of living to the full extent of one's capacities. Michel Foucault saw this development as one of the foundations of the era of biopower.[54] And perhaps it is no coincidence that, as this possibility became more important to more people, writers in the German philosophical tradition began to see death as a spur to human flourishing, as well as a limitation on it. Schopenhauer suggested that all religious and philosophical systems are in the end an antidote to 'the terrible certainty of death'.[55] Hegel went further, defining the whole of history as 'what man does with death'.[56] For Theodor Adorno, 'the simple fact must be recognised that that which is specifically cultural is that which is removed from the naked dependency of life'.[57] Culture, in his famous definition, 'is that which goes beyond the self-preservation of the species'.[58]

If death heralds the extinction of possibilities for the dying person, the pursuit of immortality seems, by contrast, to be bound up with the end of culture. Sergey Brin, one of the founders of Google, has invested over $1 billion in a 'longevity lab' called Calico (short for the California Life Company), which aims to 'make death optional'. Brin is just one among several Silicon Valley billionaires hoping not to die. If cryogenics proves to be unequal to the task, then a range of other biological tools stand ready to help defeat death: nanorobotic devices will scour the blood to cleanse it of disease and reverse the ravages of ordinary ageing; we can call on bionic limbs (and perhaps eyes and ears too); we may even be able to reformat our genes. This hyper-optimistic view of mortality has been described in detail by the Israeli historian Yuval Noah Harari in his book *Sapiens: A Brief History of Humankind* (2011). Harari predicts that average life expectancy could double this century to 150 as a result of a biotechnological revolution. Harari follows Ray Kurzweil in arguing that humans are on the cusp of ceasing to be Homo sapiens and are becoming instead 'completely different beings who possess not only different physiques, but also very different cognitive and emotional worlds'.[59] The world Harari goes on to imagine is a dystopian one in which those with the wealth to transform themselves into cyborgs control everything and the boundaries between machines, animals and social systems are held in place by data algorithms; liberal society collapses and a kind of Hobbesian *bellum omnium contra omnes* is unleashed in which untransformed humans will subsist as what some in Silicon Valley call 'meat puppets'. This seems to be a confirmation of the intuition behind so much nineteenth-century German thought on death, that it is in some sense a precondition for culture.

We could sharpen the point further and say that death exposes the hollowness of individualism. Nothing shines a light on a group's values like its response to the deaths of others. This is the meaning of Tolstoy's wonderful satire. It is still possible to develop relations with dying persons, especially in the intimate sphere (as the bond between Ivan and his servant Gerasim shows), even if Ivan Ilyich's intimates had no interest in doing so.

An important corollary of the approach to the pariah syndrome that we have set down here is that illness itself is not generally the cause of abandonment. There are situations where healthy others have a powerful biological incentive to withdraw from the sick. But this is seldom the case in WEIRD societies. Before the advent of the SARS-COV2 pandemic, infectious diseases accounted for a tiny proportion of deaths occurring in the USA, the UK and most countries in northern Europe, and most of those deaths were of elderly people suffering from flu. If members of WEIRD societies feel unsafe in the presence of the ill, it is because WEIRD cultures are unreceptive to the very idea of major illness, for reasons that go beyond biological danger. It is the *idea* of illness more than its reality that drives the healthy and the able-bodied away. That is why those with invisible conditions – as David Rabin's still was in San Marino – are just as likely to be turned into pariahs as people with visible conditions.

Coda

We have deliberately left to the end a discussion of the one theoretical trend that has addressed the pariah syndrome in detail. This is the evolutionary psychological school. We recognize that disease raises significant evolutionary challenges for any species and that there must be a place for evolutionary thinking in accounting for how humans manage it. The evolutionary psychological approach tries to find specific adaptations to explain our feelings about disease and those who carry them.

In a widely cited paper, two evolutionary psychologists, Robert Kurzban and Mark R. Leary, proposed that the human mind may contain an adaptation that causes us to avoid those with parasitic infections.[60] They argue that the avoidance of the ill may be the result of this adaptation, which is much more powerful as a motivating factor than we allow ourselves to know. They write that 'Seemingly irrational decisions with respect to knowledge that someone is infected with aids, or even cancer, might be manifestations of the operation of these hypervigilant systems.' The idea of such an adaptation is not far-fetched, but the idea of it operating independently of, and without reference to, other adaptive functions seems implausible.

A different explanation for the isolation of the ill has been offered by two other evolutionary psychologists, John Tooby and Leda Cosmides.[61] Starting off from the notion that organisms construct niches that modify their own and other organisms' niches, they point out that mammalian species in general and humans in particular are primed 'to find and occupy individualized niches that are unusually other-benefitting but hard to imitate'. We set out to make ourselves seem irreplaceable in the eyes of significant others. Tooby and Cosmides suggest that perennial complaints about feeling anonymous in modern mass societies may actually be battening off our adaptive need for confirmation of our own irreplaceability. The feeling of irreplaceability, they conjecture, enabled our hominid ancestors to bond together more tightly and to trust one another, permitting some to pursue 'more productive, but more injury producing subsistence practices, such as large game hunting'. It also helped our hominid ancestors to blunt the effect of something Tooby and Cosmides name the 'Banker's Paradox'. Bankers have a fixed amount of money to lend and usually there are plenty of would-be borrowers seeking loans. Every loan is a gamble. Often, the best strategy is to lend money to those who need it least, because they are the best credit risks, and to deprive those who need it most, because they are the worst. This is the Banker's Paradox. The experience of irreplaceability means that sometimes at least we will expend time and resources on others who, from a banker's point of view, represent a higher risk. Significantly, they think that there are very strict limits on our willingness to take this risk, and illness is one of them. Here is what they say:

> If the object of investment dies, becomes permanently disabled, leaves the social group, or experiences a permanent and debilitating social reversal, then the investment will be lost. If the trouble an individual is in increases the probability of such outcomes when compared to the prospective fortunes of other potential exchange partners, then selection might be

expected to lead to the hardhearted abandonment of those in certain types of need. In contrast, if a person's trouble is temporary or they can easily be returned to a position of full benefit-dispensing competence by feasible amounts of assistance (e.g., extending a branch to a drowning person), then personal troubles should not make someone a less attractive object of assistance.[62]

Roni Rabin speaks in terms that resonate uncannily with Tooby and Cosmides's theory. 'I hate meeting new people,' she writes. 'I hate explaining the situation anew, and I'm convinced I'll scare them off. Who'd want to get involved with such a messy situation? And what a demand to start off with, as a friend in need.'[63]

The game theory described in Tooby and Cosmides's theory captures the dilemma of individuals in WEIRD societies well enough. One might say the predictions they make about the situation of the sick and the disabled are amply borne out there. But it is less convincing as conjectural history. Humans as a species always lived in groups. Tooby and Cosmides posit an individual who is at all times seeking to maximize his or her own personal advantage. For most of our species' history this has been an impossible goal; individualism usually proved fatal. Moreover, the theory of embeddedness as a collection of evolutionary investments (rather like a stock market portfolio) doesn't advance our understanding of the healthy other's freedom in relation to illness. Indeed, it seems to assume that such freedom will be of no interest.

What both these theories neglect is the fact that humans as a species have developed socially by demonstrating inventiveness and courage in the face of adversity. As Richard Lewontin pointed out as long ago as 1983, organisms do not simply adapt to their environments;

they create them 'out of the bits and pieces of the external world'.[64] Lewontin invented the term 'ecological niches' to describe the way organisms of all kinds flexibly rework their environments in their own immediate, medium- and long-term interests and then rework them again when reversals occur. In the case of human organisms, culture is powerfully involved in this multifaceted process because the essentially symbolic meanings that come from culture are what free the human order from mere biological necessity. The rituals, beliefs and sedimented experience passed down through language, customs and folk memory open up a very wide range of possibilities for human ecological niches. The biologically based intersubjectivity on which these depend can be harnessed and refocused in countless ways. Evolutionary psychology is often more alive to the constraints placed on culture by biology than to the massive range of cultural possibilities biology enables. It could be argued that WEIRD societies have improvised an ecological niche based on forms of sociability that in some domains minimize the power of group life. These encourage us to see the body from the perspective of an atomized 'consumer' who, out of 'trained incapacity', not only seeks to steer clear of the body and its vicissitudes, but makes it, under certain circumstances, an object of utmost stigma, allowing full legitimacy to the healthy and fictionally immutable body alone. It is a niche fashioned by forms of modernity driven above all by deregulation, privatization and casualization, which in turn weaken social solidarity in all its forms, throwing the individual back on his or her own resources to an unprecedented extent while at the same depriving most individuals of the institutional support necessary to make use of those same resources. Until that changes, the isolation of the ill is destined to remain a social fact in the full Durkheimian sense, that is, a state of affairs that does not originate in the decisions made by individuals but whose presence can be recognized by its widespread diffusion in WEIRD societies and 'by the resistance offered against every individual act that tends to contravene it'. It is an example of what Durkheim called a 'pathological social fact'.[65] Another world is possible. For as Zygmunt Bauman has observed:

> The job with which humans are charged today remains much the same as it has been since the beginning of modern times: the self-constitution of individual life and the weaving as well as the servicing of the networks of bonds with other self-constituting individuals.[66]

We hope that in this chapter we have highlighted the kinds of bonds that individuals need to recreate and in many cases discover for the first time. In the next chapter we will show how these bonds determine health outcomes and the social distribution of illness.

4

Biopsychosocial Beings

Throughout this book we have paid special attention to the embeddedness of psychobiological processes in the human response to illness. These processes, we argued, were somewhat hidden in WEIRD societies, and often discounted. In the first chapter, we described emergent illness and collective attempts to normalize it by making it conform to some familiar pattern. We suggested that a great deal of normalization takes place out of awareness. Intimates, we observed, tend to pool their psychophysical resources; this often results in the healthy not noticing signs of emerging illness in a close other, or – just as striking after a diagnosis – identifying completely with their condition. Among non-intimates, the situation is more complicated. They do not pool their psychophysical capacities to the same extent. In consequence, they are often more alert to signs of emergent illness in others, which can make them fearful. In both cases, we described a dialectic of denial and acceptance (of the symptom or of the illness it may presage) that becomes more visible as the illness unfolds. We stressed that it was important not to equate denial with dysfunction or acceptance with robustness and rationality: denial, we observed, may go with resilience, while the legacy of acceptance may be heightened fear. The decisive factor is whether the healthy regard the sick other as a close other and wish to go on regarding him or her in that way. We argued that once the presence of an illness is acknowledged, there are only two possible courses of action open to healthy others: they can either care for the sick other, or they abandon him or her (perhaps on the assumption that others will step in).

The nature of care was the subject of Chapter Two. We followed Arthur Kleinman in seeing care as a general human capacity whose roots can be seen in infancy and which is shaped to a high degree by the biological, psychological and social development of the carer. Care is centrally involved in how we make the world our own and how we adapt to what we have made. Generally speaking, it arises on a foundation of mutual recognition. There are exceptions, as for example when the care recipient is so ill as to be unconscious. We nevertheless argued that in general the 'logic of care' (to use Annemarie Mol's phrase) follows the logic of intersubjective contact; that is, it is dependent on certain evolutionarily specified powerful elaborations of coordinated movement, arousal management and meaning-making. Together these combine to produce a momentum towards play, where play is understood as the pleasurable and creative use of the symbolic resources present in a relational context. Care necessarily involves a formidable amount of subject–object confusion, because it is in the nature of strong intersubjective contact to blur the boundaries of each individual's experience. And crucially, we argued that these claims about care are borne out in many professional descriptions of medical consultations.

In order to emphasize the psychobiological components of care, Chapter Two bracketed off the social world and cultural context. These were brought back into our model in Chapter Three when we considered the abandonment of the ill. We described a threshold of neurobiological synchrony that fosters group resilience in the face of all kinds of adversity, including illness and bereavement, arguing that the way to reach that threshold is through: a) public expressions of group affiliatedness; b) a group assumption that supporters of the sick person will themselves be supported; c) rituals and other activities fostering shared bodily rhythms; and d) a willingness to interpret what happens in a culturally meaningful way. These are the forms that coordinated movement, arousal management and shared meaning-making take in healthy adult life. We suggested that when we are faced with major illness the social context of contemporary modernity tends to deprive us of these props. In our discussion of ordinary embodied strangeness, we suggested that even healthy embodiment has an unsettling aspect that healthy humans typically suppress by engaging with others whom they take to be like themselves. Among intimates, this history of positive mirroring may take on a life of its own in the shape of implicit relational knowing. Implicit relational knowing might be thought of as a valuable psychobiological confirmation that we know how to be with another person. Illness, we suggested, may powerfully impair our recourse to this process. The feature of ordinary embodied strangeness that dominates our social existence is the pursuit of safety. Drawing on Stephen W. Porges's Polyvagal Theory, we argued that the pursuit of safety finds expression in neurobiological coregulation, something most of us rely upon more than we know. Finally, in that chapter we described some of the ways in which contemporary modernity makes salient and 'thematizes' certain aspects of our bodily experience while playing down some others to the point that they seem meaningless.

Our goal in this chapter is to place the argument so far in an updated version of the biopsychosocial model of health and disease. It may be helpful if we first set out the bare bones of the argument, before filling it in.

Studies in epidemiology, epigenetics and social neuroscience completed since the 1980s tell us that the history of our interpersonal engagements has a decisive, cumulative effect on human health. They indicate that social adversity can become embedded in the body physiologically, leading to greater risk of illness and death. Obviously, interpersonal engagements are not the only things that make us well or ill; biogenic causation is also real. Epistemologically, the challenge is how to explain the interplay of bottom-up causation (from the cell upwards, say) with its top-down counterpart (psychosocial experience, initiated by the environment). A number of frameworks have been developed with this end in view. Within medicine, the one that is best known is the biopsychosocial model of health and disease, first described in a series of papers by George Engel in the late 1970s and early 1980s.[1] More recent proposals include neuroecosociality, ecosociality, biocultures and developmental systems theory, though this list is far from exhaustive.[2] One of us (Derek Bolton) has recently published a monograph in the philosophy of medicine setting out the basis for a new understanding of the biopsychosocial model of health and disease, one that takes account of developments in the health sciences since Engel's papers appeared.[3] We will draw on that understanding in this chapter. Engel's biopsychosocial model is more penetrating and challenging than it is often given credit for, but he was writing before the full implications of biopsychosociality were clear. There is some overlap between the model we will present and Engel's original presentation of his model. Engel grounded his thinking in the notion of humans as nonlinear, dynamic, open biological systems, as do we. He saw regulation – the maintenance of homeostatic balance – as the fundamental task of these systems. He was also aware of the role of stressors (anything which throws a system out of homeostatic balance) and buffering (anything that blunts the effect of a stressor) in producing health and disease. In Engel's case, this trio appears in the guise of David Rosenthal's 'stress diathesis model' of schizophrenia, which Engel drew upon. The stress diathesis model hypothesized that some people had a biological predisposition or 'diathesis' that made them vulnerable to schizophrenia under conditions of stress. Engel thought the same aetiological pattern might apply to a wide variety of medical illnesses. Engel's philosophically deep critique of physicalism in medicine – the assumption, as he put it, that 'the language of chemistry and physics will ultimately suffice to explain biological phenomena' – and his powerful interrogation of the notion of 'predisposition' have largely stood the test of time.[4] But Engel lacked two further concepts which we will suggest are crucial. The first was something approximating James Gibson's notion of 'affordances' (crudely, the range of possibilities for action that a given environment offers the organism).[5] The second is the role of 'embodied agency', or what the epidemiologist Michael Marmot calls 'autonomy with support' in producing states of health and disease, a topic on which, if the sceptical reader will bear with us, we shall offer some original speculations. And perhaps most significantly of all, Engel did not really have a theory of how the organism exercises discretion over which affordances to call upon: biological, psychological or social.

The biopsychosocial model that we will present draws on all these concepts. Most of the mechanisms we have been concerned with in this book are buffering mechanisms. Normalization and holding are buffering mechanisms. The threshold of neurobiological synchrony that we described in Chapter Three is also a source of buffering. And buffering is a pivotal aspect of care of all kinds. Care is the source of our embodied agency. This is so not only in the banal, tautological sense that without care we would have little or no embodied agency, but because over time the elements of care (powerful elaborations of coordinated movement, arousal management and meaning-making) fuse to create a rich implicit sense of the self in the world. Our health is massively dependent upon this implicit self because it is the source of our embodied agency. Finally, with biopsychosociality in mind, it is obvious why infant care offers a better model of care in general than healthcare. Healthcare is concerned primarily with remedying or palliating deficits or impairments. Infant care succeeds by forming a synergistic system with a needy other to enable that other to develop their own capacities. The latter enables us to reckon with the implications of thinking of humans as open biological systems. What the health sciences since Engel have demonstrated is that when our social existence as individuals is compromised by adversity or isolation, we tend to lose coherence as organisms: achieved states of complexity break down.[6] This loss of organismic coherence is only a tendency: an increase in the probability of illness based on a wide range of exposures to different sorts of risks; but at a population level the effects of what has been called the 'exposome' are striking.[7]

Without an understanding of these things, we cannot know what illness really is as a social fact. Perhaps more importantly, we won't know what to do about it. Members of WEIRD societies behave badly around illness in part because they don't recognize the power of the collective. They think illness is largely if not exclusively a matter of biology. Or to make this point another way: they do not recognize the role of care in shaping health outcomes over the long term. The theory we have been expounding throughout this book lends strong support to a programme for political action. The way to improve health and raise life expectancy across the board is not to take two hundred pills a day, like Ray Kurzweil and his admirers in Silicon Valley, but to promote economic, civic and political equality, and a cohesive society based on the recognition of the dignity of all.

The chapter, then, will unfold as follows. In the first section, we will consider the origins of the biopsychosocial model that Engel developed. Biopsychosocial thinking was initiated by physicians.

It did not come from social science. The clinicians who were most committed to it and who tried to develop research programmes out of it thought that clinical consultations were where the model would be tested and eventually vindicated. Engel, for instance, carried out *very* long-term longitudinal studies of single patients with this aim in view. In the second section, we consider what turned out to provide the most powerful support for the biopsychosocial model: large-scale epidemiological studies – notably the Whitehall Study in the UK, the 'adverse childhood events' or ACEs study in the USA, which was reproduced around the world, and research carried out worldwide into the social determinants of health – and studies in epigenetics and social neuroscience. In our third and final section, we focus on the relationship between biopsychosociality and some of the studies in question, paying special attention to why supported autonomy and embodied agency seems to have such a determining effect on states of health.

The sources of the biopsychosocial model

By way of a prologue, it should be noted that what is and always has been at stake in the biopsychosocial model is the idea that meaningful generalizations can be made about psychosocial causation across the whole human species.[8] Since at least the ancient Greeks, Western medicine has always recognized psychosocial causation as a possibility, especially in connection with mental illnesses; what has been in doubt is how far disease processes in general can be ascribed to a psychosocial cause. Among lay people today, psychosocial causation has an odd status. It is widely thought to be selective on certain personality types, a legacy perhaps of the success of Friedman and Rosenman's concept of 'Type A personalities.'[9] Such people were said to be driven and ambitious. They were always stressed and the combination of stress and drivenness made them especially vulnerable to heart attacks. But in the folk imagination, Type A personalities were something of an exception: most illnesses were still thought to be biogenic, the result of an unhealthy lifestyle or plain bad luck in the genetic lottery. As George Engel observed in 1977, biomedicine is our folk model of how health and disease come about. We think of disease and disease states as paradigmatically biological.[10] It might sound strange to complain that most laboratory-based medical research looks for biological causes only – after all, what else would one look for in a lab? – but thanks largely to the 'big data' 'omics' disciplines of genomics, transcriptomics, proteomics and so on, we are now in a position to examine at least some of the biological traces of life experiences. This is a game-changing shift.

Occasionally, biological causes have been found that have appeared to discredit the very idea of psychosocial causation. Perhaps the most famous instance of such a cause came with the discovery of the role of *Helicobacter pylori* in peptic ulcers. For much of the twentieth century peptic ulcers were thought to be caused by psychological stress. But in the 1980s two medical students, Barry Marshall and Robin Warren, discovered that most cases of peptic ulcer were caused by *H. pylori*, as it became known.[11] Even so, only a fraction of those infected with *H. pylori* go on to develop peptic ulcer syndrome and it remains the case that psychological stress increases the risk of peptic ulcer regardless of infection.[12]

Versions of the biopsychosocial model have been circulating arguably since the 1920s. The version Engel developed had two major sources. The first was stress research, which in the English-speaking world at any rate was identified with the Harvard physiologist Walter B. Cannon (1871–1945), the discoverer of homeostasis – that is, the tendency of the body to maintain a dynamically stable state counteracting disturbances by external forces or influences.[13] The proto-biopsychosocial idea in play here was the notion that the body is in constant 'dialogue' with the environment. Cannon was a pioneer in documenting the physiological impact of psychological responses. He showed, for instance, that when the body is in shock, concentrations of sugar in the blood rise. The thirst we experience as a result of this increase enables us to dilute the concentration of sugar. This was homeostasis in action. Cannon also coined the term 'the fight–flight reaction'. This turned on the idea that the mind could trigger a volley of far-reaching physiological changes caused by the release of adrenaline into the bloodstream. These changes collectively allowed the human being to institute a different stable state better adapted to meeting the environmental challenge facing him or her at that particular moment. The other outstanding contributor to this strand of psychosomatic medicine was Hans Selye (1907–1982), through whose work the idea of stress took hold. ('Stress' was a term Cannon had imported from metallurgy.) Selye was interested in a wide-ranging response of the animal body to what he initially termed 'generalized unpleasantries'. It was Selye who gave the name 'stressor' to anything that disturbs homeostatic balance. Selye was the first person to demonstrate the role of the whole endocrine system in generating the set of somatic reactions which we know today as the stress response. The stress response was mediated by what he called the 'pituitary adrenal axis'. He believed that, in the end, repeated adaptation to stress led to disease. He thought stress resulted in disease because humans ran out of the hormones necessary to sustain the adaptation, especially adrenaline (a hypothesis we now know to be false).[14]

Psychoanalysis was the other source of inspiration for Engel's vision. The key figure here was Franz Alexander (1891–1964) who in

1932 set up the Chicago Institute of Psychoanalysis, independently of the American Psychoanalytic Association. Unlike every other psychoanalytic institute in the world, the Chicago Institute was not specifically focused on mental health. Instead, trainees were invited to study the role of psychic factors, especially recurrent emotions, in *bodily* disturbances. Alexander and his collaborators Therese Benedek and Helen Flanders Dunbar popularized the idea that certain kinds of disorders went with certain kinds of personality types, a notion that held sway until quite recently through the concept of Type A personalities. They hypothesized, for example, that chronic inhibition of rage led to high blood pressure. Chronicity was a sign that the rage was longstanding and possibly infantile in origin. The overlap between the American psychoanalytic version of psychosomatic medicine and the vision of Cannon, Selye and the stress researchers lay in the fact that both were firmly rooted in a holistic conception of the total human organism responding dynamically to various stimuli, threats and assaults from the environment.

George Engel began his career as a general physician in a hospital with a strong interest in stress research and was for many years hostile to psychoanalysis. But under the influence of John Romano and others he trained at the Chicago Institute.[15] Though he remained a critical friend of psychoanalysis for the rest of his life, the research he carried out in psychosomatic medicine focused on the relationship between very basic psychological experiences and physiological changes. With his colleague Franz Reichsman, Engel was involved for over forty years in the treatment of a patient he called Monica.[16] Monica was born with an oesophageal atresia, a blockage in the tube connecting her mouth to her stomach, and had to be fed through a fistula that was inserted into her stomach. Monica's nineteen-year-old mother found it hard to bond with her daughter (partly because she could not feed her in the normal way), and mother and daughter were also subjected to periods of enforced separation caused by Monica's numerous hospitalizations. When Monica was fifteen months old she was admitted to hospital, where she stayed for some nine months, during which time she became attached to Reichsman and one of the nurses, both of whom in turn became attached to her. Engel observed that during periods of separation from these figures, Monica never cried but became unresponsive and withdrawn. Her muscle tone decreased; she became very still and looked sad. Most worrying of all, her gastric secretions ceased (which meant that she couldn't digest food). Whenever Reichsman or the nurse reappeared, Monica's muscle tone returned; she moved about, showed joy and her gastric secretion rates increased. Engel and Reichsman named the complex of psychophysiological withdrawal a 'depression-withdrawal reaction'. Graeme Taylor, a liaison psychiatrist who trained with Reichsman, recalled that the two men believed that 'hidden within the interactions between infant and mother are a number of processes by which the mother serves as an external regulator not only of the infant's behaviour and autonomic physiology, but also of the neurochemistry of its maturing brain.'[17] In many respects, Engel's and Reichman's Monica studies are consilient with modern attachment theory, which emphasizes attachment's role in promoting buffering. The 'depression-withdrawal reaction' invites comparison with a homologous distinction in Bowlby's attachment theory which emphasized the far-reaching biological consequences of moving from what he called 'protest' to 'despair' or 'giving up.'[18] Giving up is what leads to chronic depression in Bowlby's system. And Engel, like Bowlby, took care to distinguish depression-withdrawal from psychological melancholia of the kind described by Freud, which was essentially about conflict *with* another rather than the need *for* another. Engel thought that depression-withdrawal could be seen across the life cycle and wanted to investigate if it might be an important predisposing factor in bringing about physical disease.

Engel was aware that the biological, the psychological and the social did not interact in ways that affected everyone in the same way. About diabetes, for instance, he says this:

> the biochemical defect constitutes but one factor among many, the complex interaction of which ultimately may culminate in active disease or manifest illness. Nor can the biochemical defect be made to account for all of the illness, for full understanding requires additional concepts and frames of reference. Thus, while the diagnosis of diabetes is first suggested by certain core clinical manifestations, for example, polyuria, polydipsia, polyphagia, and weight loss, and is then confirmed by laboratory documentation of relative insulin deficiency, how these are experienced and how they are reported by anyone individual, and how they affect him, all require consideration of psychological, social, and cultural factors, not to mention other concurrent or complicating biological factors.[19]

Similarly, a holistic framework was required to take account of psychological and social factors. Only some people would respond as Monica had to separation from a carer, just as only some people would respond to 'the demands of the social system in which they are living and working' by becoming ill. The challenge, as Engel saw it, was to lay new conceptual foundations for medical science that would explain individual differences. Biomedicine offered a very succinct answer: they were ultimately rooted in bodily differences. Biomedicine was committed to physicalism, the notion that biological systems are physical in nature, and reductionism, the philosophic view that complex phenomena are ultimately derived from a single primary principle. On this view, the single primary principle to which all disease could be traced was molecular biology, which was understood to rest on the laws of physics. Engel also insisted that the biomedical model was based on mind–body dualism because it treated the mind and the body as distinct and separable.[20] The task he set himself in his landmark paper of 1977 was to deepen the theoretical and scientific foundations of medical practice in a way that would make room for the possibility of psychosocial causation and at the same time shed light on the question of why humans do not respond identically to the same biological, psychological and social challenges.

David Rosenthal's stress-diathesis model supplied a useful starting point. As already mentioned, Rosenthal had conjectured that some people had a biological predisposition or 'diathesis' that made them vulnerable to schizophrenia under conditions of stress.[21] Although Rosenthal was focused on a single psychiatric disorder, here *in embryo* was the notion of gene–environment interaction: a disorder with a genetic basis could be amplified by the environment in which a person develops.

Rosenthal's idea was taken up by the American psychiatrist Seymour Kety. Kety led an important study, the Danish–American Schizophrenia Study. This study made the first attempt to demonstrate the possibility of gene–environment interaction in the evolution of schizophrenia. Rosenthal was a co-investigator on the later parts of the study. The study was carried out in Denmark because the Danish government held full details of the biological and adoptive families of all adoptions that had taken place on Danish soil since 1924. This information could be linked to hospital data on admissions to hospital for mental health conditions. Kety and his colleagues examined a cohort of 5,500 adoptees living in or around Copenhagen. They looked at the incidence of psychiatric conditions in the adoptive families and the biological families of some 34 adoptees who had received a diagnosis of schizophrenia.[22] These 34 patients were then matched to 33 controls with no history of psychiatric illness. The researchers tracked down medical records on 463 relatives of the 67 index cases (the 34 adoptees with a diagnosis of schizophrenia and the 33 controls) and these were examined by four Danish psychiatrists. They found more schizophrenic relatives among the schizophrenic adoptees than among the controls. But they also found that adoptees were more likely to meet the diagnostic criteria for schizophrenia if one or both of their adoptive parents had the disorder. This suggested that socially mediated psychological experience could amplify a biological effect significantly. The bio, the psycho and the social could produce synergies that were not reducible to the bio.

When Engel came to formulate his own version of the bio-psychosocial model of health and disease in the late 1970s, it was precisely this sort of interaction that he had in mind. And he turned to Kety and through him to Rosenthal for support. His first paper on the biopsychosocial model drew heavily on Kety's work. In spite of Engel's reservations about the use of full psychoanalysis in medical treatments, his psychoanalytic sympathies were sufficiently well known that he feared his model would be seen as a kind of 'psychoanalysis by the back door'. Kety was known to be hostile to psychoanalysis and his credentials as a biological psychiatrist were unimpeachable. Kety had also published a paper outside the framework of the Danish–American Schizophrenia Study in which he suggested that a different diathesis might explain diabetes.[23] Factors which by themselves might have little or no impact on health or illness could in combination with others become pathogenic.

Engel could not demonstrate this possibility *in vivo* for other conditions, but he could represent it by appealing to the notion of open biological systems that Ludwig von Bertalanffy, the originator of systems theory, had formulated in the late 1940s.[24] Open systems are systems that exchange matter and energy with the environment. Open biological systems can stave off the entropy or decay suffered by physical systems by maintaining themselves in a high state of order (that is, capable of transitioning to a higher state of complexity) by drawing sustenance of various kinds from the environment and expelling waste. It was an axiom of systems theory that open systems could not be described in mechanistic terms. Instead, the key idea was that the state of an open system at any given moment was *flexibly determined* by any or all of the causal powers acting upon it. This meant that the relationships among causal factors were not law-like.

Biological, psychological and social events operated according to different timescales. And within each category there was also wide variation. Roughly speaking, the more complex the system, the longer the timeframe. Neurophil cells last only two days but the cells in our eye lenses last a lifetime. Generally speaking, most of the cells in our bodies last between seven and ten years. A child is born with a relatively undeveloped left brain. The organs age at different paces. But Engel makes nothing of this fact. Because he misses time, Engel also misses development. Everything is assumed to be fully formed, from subatomic particles upwards. Yet if we think about children, say, as open biological systems, we are soon confronted with the fact that a baby's nervous system is different from a toddler's, which in turn is different from an adult's. This changes the kinds of information the developing human will exchange with its environment. Sometimes, in order to transition to a higher level of complexity and coherence, children have to undo some of the development that enabled them to reach the previous stage. A toddler about to walk must give up crawling, for example. The environment still has to enable the infant to receive the right combination of supports if she is to move on to the next stage. Now, in fact, the more we adopt a life-course perspective, the clearer it becomes that human development turns on *emergent* biological, psychological and social capacities that transform the way the organism functions at different moments in time. The sources of these capacities are widely distributed inside and outside the body and this enables the agent to fall back on a large set of possibilities. In the terms of Ilya Prigogine and Isabelle Stengers, this is evidence of the self-organizing capacities of humans as open biological systems.[25]

Engel also lacked a sense of the sheer range of possibilities that the bio, the psycho and the social offered humans. In his wonderful online introduction to systems biology, the Israeli biologist Uri Alon describes a famous experiment by Jacques Monod carried out in the 1960s. Monod found that if you put an E. coli cell into a beaker of water and add some salt and some sugar, it will create copies of itself with astonishing accuracy within half an hour.[26] If you place some sugar a metre or two away, the E. coli cell will undergo a complete transformation. It will create an electric motor with a propeller and a navigation system that tells it where to go to find the sugar. It will also improvise a 'pump' to enable it to extract the sugar and break it down into carbon atoms. How does it do this? A single-celled organism such as E. coli contains around three hundred transcription factor proteins that enable it to form a 'picture' of its environment. If sugar is detected, a vast array of biological transformations occurs. E. coli changes its composition according to the environment in which it finds itself. Under circumstance *a* (no sugar except in the beaker of water) it does not need to improvise any of the biological characteristics we have just described. Circumstance *b* (in which sugar is detected in the environment) triggers these other events. It is the transcription factor proteins that detect the sugar which causes the bacterial DNA to create new proteins that establish the motor, the propeller, the navigation system and the pump. The single cell has around three hundred degrees of freedom (corresponding to the three hundred transcription factors) that are tasked with representing many more degrees of freedom in the external world. How much more complex is the representation of reality in organisms such as the human body, which contain billions of cells?

The notion that biology is ultimately rooted in physics does not take account of the role of information transfer in the development of living organisms. The genetic code, for instance, translates information contained within genetic material into proteins of various sorts that ultimately enable organisms to assume a particular form and to discharge particular biological functions. There are rules governing which protein-making process to initiate, when the process should start or stop (which genes should get switched on and off) and how it should behave in the face of multiple environmental conditions. The functional variation made possible by the behavioural repertoire of even a small number of chromosomes is immense.

The action of neurotransmitters in the brain illustrates the same point in a different currency. Action potentials sweep over the terminals of neurons, triggering the release of neurotransmitters into the synapse. When these eventually reach the next neuron, they initiate a specific transient reaction. A single neuron can initiate dozens of action potentials of varying intensities that trigger different reactions. This allows for great complexity in the information that gets passed from one neuron to the next. These are just two examples of how current biological models include both biochemistry, subject to physico-chemical energy equations, *plus* models of information-based regulatory control mechanisms.

The crucial point is that regulatory control is a type of causation. To be sure, this causation is embedded in the physical properties of the organism, but the outcomes it gives rise to are sensitive to a vast range of processes occurring both inside and outside the organism, as Monod's example of the E. coli cell shows. Another way of putting this would be to say that living systems exploit the *slack* within physical laws. They take advantage of the full range of possibilities present in their own physiology in interaction with its environment. We readily think of living organisms as having subsystems that cause particular organs and functions to develop at specific times and in specific sites. Sexual differentiation, to take one example, occurs in the womb through the action of specific genetic and hormonal influences. We are perhaps slower to realize that this general feature of development leads to a dizzying array of possible outcomes within multiple nested and interacting hierarchies, with pressures coming both from the bottom up (that is, from the most fundamental subsystems of the organism itself) and from the top down (from the environment). And, as the behavioural biologist Robert M. Sapolsky has observed, 'the more genomically complex the organism, the greater the percentage of the genome devoted to gene regulation by the environment.'[27]

From an open biological systems theory viewpoint, this slack plays a crucial part in the exchange of matter and information with the environment that is essential for open biological systems. And even in the case of single-celled organisms, it is clear that these exchanges transform biology. The E. coli cell that improvises a motor, propeller, navigation system and pump is physically distinct from one that doesn't. Prigogine and Stengers would say that the former has taken a leap into a new, more differentiated, higher level of 'order' or organization. The alternative was to not reproduce itself at all or to make fewer copies of itself.

There is no reason to exclude the social and the psychological from this basic work of harnessing the environment. Both have causal effects on human health, as we will show in the next section. It is at this point that Gibson's notion of *affordances* comes into its own. Gibson defined an affordance as 'what things furnish, for good or ill'. As already mentioned, affordances alter the range of possibilities for action that a given environment offers the organism. Sugar nearby is an affordance for E. coli bacteria. School is an affordance for children enabling them to develop their minds and their social effectiveness. As Bolton and Gillett put it:

> The transition from the biological to the psychological and the social is characterised by the appearance of new free spaces in which can arise the twin phenomena of new forms of organisation and diversity and with them new causal processes. Once we move above physics and chemistry into biology, hence into psychological and social processes, the causation involves information-exchange, communication, regulation and control.[28]

States of health and disease rest on the exploitation of multiple affordances at every level of the organism's existence. They seldom have single causes. Under conditions of multilevel, dynamic, open interactions, outcomes are not fixed but will often tend in certain directions. This is something that large-scale epidemiological studies are best placed to show.

Psychosocial causation and the physiological embedding adversity

We can now say with certainty that psychosocial causation is real. Large-scale epidemiological studies tell us so. In the mid-1960s the British government agreed to fund a study looking at individual risk factors for cardiorespiratory disease and diabetes using a prospective cohort of middle-aged male British civil servants.[29] The study was called the Whitehall Study and is known today as 'Whitehall I'. Back then, coronary heart disease was assumed to result from a more affluent lifestyle and from stress, so the researchers expected to find more coronary heart disease in the senior grades, where salaries were higher and responsibilities were heavier. In fact, the very opposite proved to be the case: the lower the civil service grade, the higher the risk of death from coronary heart disease and from diabetes.[30] When the Whitehall researchers looked at all-cause mortality in the same cohort ten years later, they found the same gradient.[31] The lower the civil service grade, the higher the incidence of death from all causes. What made these findings even more surprising was that the highest levels of blood plasma cholesterol (believed to cause heart attacks) were found in the higher grades. The Whitehall Study was the first to find that social class was a risk factor in its own right for the most common causes of death. Before Whitehall, risk factors were always assumed to result from disordered somatic processes, including the stress response. When social class figured at all in epidemiological studies it was as 'a potential confounder that you got rid of in order to arrive at the "correct" conclusion about the association between risk factor and disease'.[32]

At this point the investigators decided to set up a new study known as 'Whitehall II' under the leadership of Michael Marmot.

Whitehall II recruited over 10,000 civil servants (6,895 men and 3,413 women). The gradient in health proved just as robust as it had been in the first study. Marmot and his team found

> an inverse association between employment grade and prevalence of angina, electrocardiogram evidence of ischaemia, and symptoms of chronic bronchitis. Self-perceived health status and symptoms were worse in subjects in lower status jobs. There were clear employment-grade differences in health-risk behaviours including smoking, diet, and exercise.[33]

But they also found that significant differences in 'economic circumstances, in possible effects of early-life environment as reflected by height and birth weight, in social circumstances at work (for example, monotonous work characterised by low control and low satisfaction), and in social supports.' In addition to a massive array of behavioural and biomedical variables, the researchers in Whitehall II also considered the impact of psychosocial variables on health outcomes. These included psychological workload, control over work pacing and content of work, the opportunity to use one's skills, and social support at work and at home. They considered the areas the civil servants lived in, their level of education and even the level of their parents' education. Marmot and his colleagues found that the lower the level of control over work, the greater the risk of developing coronary heart disease and minor (nonpsychotic) psychiatric disorder.[34] They also found that the combination of high efforts and low rewards predicted higher levels of coronary heart disease. Low control was a major part of the explanation of the social gradient in depressive symptoms.[35] Finally, they began to look at a subject that has proved crucial in more recent research: the buffering effect of social relationships on disease exposures.

The sheer range of data considered in Whitehall II and the number of confounding variables it took into account has made it the benchmark study for occupational cohorts worldwide.[36] It was used as a starting point in the World Health Organization's Commission on the Social Determinants of Health, which began work in 2006 under Michael Marmot's chairmanship, whose report was published in 2008.

The health gradient brought to light by Whitehall I had not previously been identified. In all WEIRD societies (and in most others too), there is a health gradient. The richer you are, the healthier you're likely to be. Perhaps there is nothing shocking about that. It is universally accepted that poverty affects health. What is surprising, though, is that if you divide populations up into socioeconomic deciles (or tenths) you will find that the richest decile is healthier than the second-richest decile, which in turn is healthier than the third richest, and so on. Today in the UK, for instance, men in the most affluent 10 per cent of the population live nine and a half years longer than men in the most deprived 10 per cent. For women, the gap is a little over seven years. If we look at *health* expectancy figures, that is, the number of disability-free life years a person can expect, the gap widens. Overall, those in the top 10 per cent experience nineteen more years of healthy life than those in the bottom 10 per cent. But surprisingly, we even find differences at the top of the scale. The top 10 per cent experiences about an extra year of life and of healthy life compared to the second richest.[37]

The question arises: why is a gradient found even among the affluent?[38] After all, in most WEIRD societies, poverty ceases three or four deciles up the scale. Lifestyle, circumstantial and behavioural factors have obvious relevance: the incidence of smoking, poor diet and alcohol consumption is known to be higher lower down the scale. But if we just focus on the top two deciles, the differences in smoking, diet and alcohol consumption are unlikely to explain the differences in health.

The gradient can't be explained in biological terms alone. We see this especially clearly in WEIRD societies. It will be recalled that Whitehall II controlled for a wide variety of lifestyle factors, as well as disparities in the possible effects of early-life environment as reflected by height and birth weight, but still found that the gradient held up. The WHO Commission looked at all member states of the WHO and found that the major discrepancies in health outcomes

> were caused by the unequal distribution of power, income, goods, and services, globally and nationally, the consequent unfairness in the immediate, visible circumstances of people's lives – their access to health care, schools, and education, their conditions of work and leisure, their homes, communities, towns, or cities – and their chances of leading a flourishing life. This unequal distribution of health-damaging experiences is not in any sense a 'natural' phenomenon but is the result of a toxic combination of poor social policies and programmes, unfair economic arrangements, and bad politics.[39]

How do psychosocial factors produce such powerful effects on health? Perhaps the most important way is via the stress response, as Cannon and Selye realized. The stress response produces system-wide effects throughout the human body. Entire books have been written about the impact of stress on the heart, the immune system, reproduction, foetal development, and child and adolescent development.[40] We will focus here, briefly, on the 'basics' of the stress response, which operates through the so-called HPA axis (hypothalamus-pituitary-adrenaline).[41] When we trigger the stress response we set off a cascade of glucocorticoids. These substances, which include cortisol, adrenaline and noradrenaline, have the effect of thickening our blood, which facilitates the forming of clots, which in turn reduces blood loss. They also raise our blood pressure, which distends the blood vessels. This distension causes the heart muscles to get bigger, which makes the blood vessels more rigid, which leads to tearing, inflammation and narrowing of the arteries. Chronic activation of the stress response results in chronically elevated blood pressure. Eventually, deposits of atherosclerotic plaque form, which act as a sponge for fat, glucose and cholesterol. One of the most striking and unexpected findings of the first Whitehall study was that senior civil servants had higher levels of cholesterol than their colleagues lower down the hierarchy but still experienced less coronary heart disease. The stress response offers a clue as to why. Cholesterol is most damaging when there is inflammation in the heart. The civil servants in the higher grades may have consumed more cholesterol but they were less stressed and it did them less harm.

The stress response has been shown to have dramatic and lasting effects if it is triggered too often early in life. Early patterns of stress activation appear to set the course for the stress response across the life cycle. Intrauterine stressors such as drugs, alcohol and maternal stress hormones can lead to a variety of diseases later on in life. Postnatal stress in the form of extreme and unpredictable situations is associated with a blunted cortisol response and with hypervigilant and/or dissociative responses. Expectations of ill-treatment shape relations with others. But the system-wide bodily consequences of chronic activation of the stress response seems to result in major illness.

Because of the determining impact of early life stress, the WHO Commission rightly took a life-course approach, emphasizing the value of, among other things, parental support, good early education opportunities, meaningful, well-paid work, decent housing and relationally rich environments. These are the social determinants of health. To be deprived of them significantly increases the risk of illness. Some of this risk is directly attributable to lifestyle and behavioural factors. But the stress response is one of the factors that seems to result in adversity becoming embedded in the bodies of those it afflicts.

The Adverse Childhood Experiences (ACE) Study, carried out in Kaiser Permanente's Department of Preventive Medicine in San Diego, in collaboration with the U.S. Centers for Disease Control and Prevention (CDC), invited around 26,000 insurees in Kaiser's health plans from the San Diego area to participate in a study of the impact of adverse childhood experiences (before the age of eighteen) on adult health. After exclusions, they were left with a cohort of over 17,000 patients in 1998.[42] The principal investigators of the study, Dr Vincent J. Felitti and Dr Robert Anda, described their study sample as 'solidly middle class' (they were rich enough to afford private health insurance at a time when over 40 million of their fellow citizens had none). The ten categories of adverse childhood experience were these: 1) emotional abuse (recurrent threats, humiliation); 2) physical abuse (beating, not spanking); 3) sexual abuse involving physical contact; 4) mother treated violently; 5) living in the same household as an alcoholic or a drug user; 6) living in a household where one or more members were imprisoned; 7) living in a household where one or more members were chronically depressed, suicidal, mentally ill or in a psychiatric hospital; 8) not being raised by both biological parents; 9) physical neglect; and 10) emotional neglect. Each participant was given an ACE score, being a count of the number of categories of adverse experience that were reported. If a study subject reported two members of their childhood household had gone to jail, that still added just one to the ACE score. There was no further scoring for multiple instances of the same category. They then correlated ACE scores against a range of common conditions. Studies like the ACE study have often been carried out on patients treated for mental health issues. And like their precursors, Felitti and Anda reported a strong correlation between childhood adversity and a history of suffering from depression, alcoholism, drug addiction and teen pregnancy or paternity. What made the ACE study unusual was its inclusion of physical conditions such as strokes, cancer, ischaemic heart disease, chronic obstructive pulmonary disorder and a range of autoimmune dysfunctions. Nine out of ten categories of ACEs significantly increased the risk of ischaemic heart disease 1.3- to 1.7-fold versus persons with no ACEs. People with an ACE score of 6 or higher died nearly twenty years earlier on average than those with a score of zero. There is now a vast medical literature addressing the neurobiological effects of early life stress on development and a number of models have been constructed to explain results like those reported by Felitti and Anda.

Now, of course ACE scores leave out a number of other factors that affect health and illness. Notoriously, they take at best only indirect account of the social determinants of health; having a parent who has spent time in prison is likely to be correlated with low socioeconomic status but many of the other ACEs are not obviously associated with the social determinants. ACE scores do not measure the quality of the *total* relational environment in which children grow up, yet one of the most important findings of the last fifteen to twenty years has been that having *some* strong relationships moderates the impact of ACEs.[43]

Recently the Dunedin Multidisciplinary Health and Development Study, one of the most intensive studies of human development we have, with over fifty years of extremely detailed data on just under a thousand research subjects, found that people who had ACE scores of 4 or higher tended to *underestimate* the number of ACEs they had experienced.[44] Finally, because ACEs were designed to capture the whole of childhood and adolescence, they take no account of the *timing* of the adversity. This is a huge omission. The building up of a baby's brain depends on what has rightly been called 'an extraordinary set and sequence of developmental and environmental experiences that influence the expression of the genome'.[45] As we have seen, it is a sequence that is extremely vulnerable to stress.

This has been shown most clearly in research into animal genomics. Take for instance rhesus monkeys. Like humans, they are born with either a long or a short version of the serotonin transporter gene (5-HTLLP). Stephen Suomi and his colleagues at the National Institute of Child Health and Human Development (NICHD) in Bethesda, Maryland, looked at the impact of mothering on serotonin metabolism in a large group of over four hundred rhesus monkeys. Half of the monkeys had been separated at birth from their mothers and been reared by their peers. The other half were left with their mothers. At six months, the peer-reared group were returned to their mothers. When the monkeys were eight years old, Suomi and his colleagues identified the version of the serotonin transporter gene that each monkey carried. They found that peer-reared monkeys with the shorter version of the gene had poorer serotonin metabolism than monkeys with the longer version, but mother-reared monkeys with the short version did just as well as those with the longer version. In other words, good mothering appears to ensure that monkeys with the shorter version of the gene still metabolize serotonin properly. This 'maternal buffering' (as it is called) is an eminently biopsychosocial example of a gene–environment interaction. With aggression it's even more interesting. Monkeys with the short version of the serotonin transporter gene were more aggressive than monkeys with the longer version, but mother-reared monkeys with the short version were the least aggressive of all. The pattern prevails in respect of alcohol consumption. Monkeys with the short version of the serotonin transporter gene were more likely to drink alcohol to excess than monkeys with the longer version, but mother-reared monkeys with the short version were less likely to drink alcohol to excess than mother-reared monkeys with the long version of the gene. In all these cases, what may be a genetic risk factor for individuals with poor early experience may actually be a genetic advantage in individuals with good early experience.[46]

How applicable might this animal research be to humans? For some time, researchers looking at human mental health looked for associations between the two variants (alleles) of the serotonin transporter gene and major mental health conditions. In the Dunedin Longitudinal study Avshalom Caspi and colleagues demonstrated that humans with the shorter version of the gene were more likely to suffer from depression than those with the longer version but only if they had higher levels of concurrent stress or if they had a history of being maltreated.[47]

Embodied agency, supported autonomy
and health inequalities

There is an important overlap in the messages coming from these very different fields. They all point to the calamitous consequences for health of restrictions on agency. If we look at the particular ACEs that Felitti and Anda selected, we find they all involve either experiencing at first hand, or witnessing someone else experience, a sudden or brutal restriction on agency. Recurrent threats and humiliation, physical and sexual abuse, and physical and emotional neglect amount to direct restrictions on agency. Living in a household where one or more members was imprisoned, or was chronically depressed, suicidal, mentally ill or in a psychiatric hospital, constitute indirect restrictions on agency. Research into the social determinants of health tells us that if you live somewhere that makes you feel unsafe, where there are no opportunities to take part in social life, where schools are poorly resourced and meaningful, adequately paid work is scarce, your risk of developing a range of major illnesses increases significantly. All of these impediments amount to restriction on agency. Biology, too, can place restrictions on our agency. In addition to all the constraints that illness and disability impose, epigenetics studies tell us that adversity can affect gene expression right across the genome.

If restrictions on agency make us ill, supported autonomy makes us well. It creates and sustains health. Humans require an environment that supports their participation in the social world. We have already seen how the most affluent decile enjoys more than nineteen extra years of healthy life compared with the most deprived decile in the UK. The well-to-do enjoy more direct control over their lives, their goals are less constrained by others and they can buy a great deal of personal and social support. Significant though these things are, status by itself appears to have an impact on health. Michael Marmot describes a study carried out by Donald Redelmeier and Sheldon Singh, who compared the life expectancies of 72 years' worth of Oscar-winning actors with those of their co-stars and with fellow Oscar nominees. Oscar winners lived four years longer than their co-stars and the actors nominated who did not win. These groups were well matched for age, sex and wealth. The extra years of life seem to have resulted from the status of being an Academy Award winner. They have more embodied agency and their autonomy is supported to a greater extent.

Take another example. Unemployment is bad for health. In the 1980s, using a sample comprising 1 per cent of the UK population identified in the 1971 national census, John Fox demonstrated that people who became unemployed experienced 20 per cent higher mortality than people who remained in work at the same social class level – a finding that has been regularly reproduced ever since. Job insecurity is also associated with poorer health outcomes. It has been established repeatedly that marriage has a beneficial effect on the health of both men and women, offering protection against a range of diseases.[48] Marriage is a major source of social support. In what have become classic studies on loneliness, John T. Cacioppo and Steven Cole demonstrated a link between having no one to confide in and gene expression. They compared blood samples of people with no confidant with others who had one or more. In the former group they found increased vascular resistance, higher systolic blood pressure, more active stress hormones, under-expression of genes with anti-inflammatory properties, over-expression of genes with pro-inflammatory properties and lower overall immunity. They also reported higher rates of mental illness.

It is likely that the benefits of social connectedness that we have been describing in this section operate within the organism in multiple ways that operate across the long, medium and short terms. Support for this idea can be found in the data on the health effects of bereavement. Widowers and widows are at risk for higher morbidity and mortality than the general population. The additional mortality risk has been found to be between 15 per cent and 20 per cent over the long term but is much higher in the period immediately following the bereavement (compared with expected mortality using standardized actuarial life tables). Some estimate that the additional risk of dying in the year following the loss of a spouse is 90 per cent higher. There are also short-term benefits of social connectedness. Holding a partner's hand releases oxytocin, which lowers cortisol levels and blood pressure.

Health and disease are to a very large extent the outcomes of the peculiar pattern of stressors and buffering factors characteristic of the individual's life. Amartya Sen, a Nobel Prize-winning economist and one of the original members of the WHO Commission on the Social Determinants of Health, famously remarked that it is not only what you have that makes you well or ill, it is also what you can *do* with what you have.[49] This is the basis of his 'capabilities' approach to health. We suggest that what Sen calls 'what you can do' is highly dependent on the extent to which others support your autonomy. None of this is to deny the strong role of biology in determining health outcomes. If we turn to the research in animal and human epigenetics on the serotonin transporter gene, we will surely be compelled to acknowledge that some biological dispositions are also intrinsically buffering.

Biomedicine has no principled, scientific way of taking account of the impact of psychosocial causation. It assumes that in order to explain health, one need appeal only to the organism's own biological nature, which is conceived of in fairly static terms. The idea that the organism is constantly modifying its own biological nature, by manipulating an environment that acts upon it, is absent, except in relation to things that act biochemically: for example, an alcoholic giving himself or herself liver disease by continuing to drink alcohol. Biomedicine can only take biological insults into account. By contrast, what the biopsychosocial medical sciences show us is that social and psychological experiences also have a decisive effect on health. It is impossible to determine in advance how a particular person will respond to the total set of environmental challenges that confront a person, whether they will use the affordances at their disposal to move towards a more coherent state or towards entropy. It is precisely because of the sheer variety of biological and environmental affordances that individuals do not respond in the same way to the same external pressures.

How might the biopsychosocial model presented in skeleton form in the first part of this chapter shed light on these phenomena? We think that infant research – that most biopsychosocial field – offers some vital clues.

Children are born into a world full of meanings. The doyen of child psychologists Jerome Bruner points out that culture enables the intentional structure underlying those meanings to be deciphered.[50] From a developmental point of view, the most significant affordances shaping babies', and later toddlers', lives are cultural. Usually, by the time they are nine or ten months old, they develop an interest in marking out the distinction between the exceptional and the ordinary. Showing they understand this difference is one of the chief ways in which they mark their entry into that culture. They become familiar with songs like 'Ring a ring of roses' or they play the peep-o game, both of which play with expectations and the suspension of expectations. Their agentive self is born. '*I* was the one who covered my face so you thought I'd vanished,' they seem to say, 'and *my* perspective on the game we've just been playing is the authoritative one.' Social meanings are the main form of information that humans exchange with their environments. Without a public identity that signals to others that we have agency, our capacity to share meanings with others is very limited.

Bruner thinks that we need to be able to talk about our embodied agency because embodied agency is something we have to negotiate with others. If we can talk about our perspective *on* the world *to* the world, we may acquire a degree of mastery over it. This process is intrinsically buffering. The alternative is indefinite conflict. Bruner calls our use of this process our narrative capacity. Narrative capacity in Bruner's system is what we rely on to account for and control the meanings we want to share with the world.

The primary function of narrative in Bruner's system is to mitigate the conflicts that 'threaten breaches in the ordinariness of life'. As conflicts arise, children need to be able to say what happened, who did it, how they did it, whether it was right that they did it and how they feel about it. It is this situation that narrative is designed to address. Narratives deal with the very

> stuff of human action and human intentionality. It mediates between the canonical world of culture and the more idio-syncratic world of beliefs, desires, and hopes . . . It reiterates the norms of the society without being didactic. And . . . it provides a basis for rhetoric without confrontation. It can even teach, conserve memory, or alter the past.[51]

'Stories,' according to Bruner, 'make "reality" a mitigated reality.' This is a subtle point, but it is full of resonance for our argument because

Bruner is saying that the narrative understanding that comes through meaningful negotiation of experience in the world with others *buffers* us, perhaps at a very low level, but more or less constantly.

What happens when our narrative purchase on the world is invalidated, when we cannot measure up to our culture's notions of what an agentive self should be? We become cut off from the world of meanings. We lose some or all of this buffering. In Bertalanffy's or in Prigogine and Stenger's terms, the primary desideratum of open biological systems – to exchange matter and information with the environment – becomes constrained.

The term meanings, rather like the term narrative, highlights the role of the mind in such exchanges – possibly a little too much. Ed Tronick, some of whose work we discussed in Chapters Two and Three, was one of Bruner's most distinguished collaborators. Tronick has tried to expand the nature of the meanings in question to encompass more of their physiological correlates. He specifically says that meaning itself needs to be reconceived in biopsychosocial terms. Tronick suggests that when a preverbal infant finds a way of connecting with the people and things around him, he experiences a 'state of consciousness'. States of consciousness are psychobiological. They tell us about our 'sense of self and our place in the world'.[52] They are not the sole preserve of infants; they are also the basic building blocks of adult mental life. Tronick invites us to imagine how we as adults feel when we're in an aeroplane that is hit by turbulence. Most of us have a multi-layered experience in that situation. We may think to ourselves 'this turbulence is unpleasant, I wish it would stop.' But that thought will be accompanied by all manner of physiological, neurological, endocrine and other somatic states. States of consciousness surpass ordinary cognitive awareness by including these states. When we make a judgement about how much agency we can exercise in the world – in the plane hit by turbulence, for example – we initiate a range of processes that involve the whole body. These are action-based, often rooted in direct experimental attempts to reckon with the possible. They are dynamic and involve feedback loops. And they are multimodal, comprising, inter alia, sensory inputs, cognition, motor planning and perhaps even something like a psychodynamic unconscious, all fundamentally in the service of action in the environment.

Now, the most important thing about states of consciousness in Tronick's system is that they take account of the biological undergirding of Bruner's cultural 'meanings'. Tronick suggests that there are three main ways in which states of consciousness can expand in complexity and coherence. Adults can engage with their states of consciousness through introspection. They might wonder if they're wrong to be so disturbed by a bit of turbulence. They can also take an interest in the relationship between the experiences at the heart of the state of consciousness and the world of things. They can console themselves that planes are built for turbulence and try to reimmerse themselves in whatever they were doing before the turbulence. But the most immediately powerful way to strengthen a state of consciousness is by forming an intersubjective system with another person and using the experience of that psychobiological relationship to regulate the state of consciousness. They can turn to their neighbour in the next seat and laugh together about their surprisingly panicky reaction. As we saw in Chapter Two, Tronick calls this process 'dyadic consciousness'. Strong states of dyadic consciousness are characterized by what Tronick calls 'impelling certitudes', and are underpinned by a coherence of physiology, feeling, action and thought about one's self and one's relationship with others and the world.[53] It is possible that something like impelling certitudes are relevant to the processes that eventually manifest in the health gradient.

An interesting corollary of Tronick's theory is that some forms of dyadic consciousness can be profoundly obstructive if we form intersubjective systems with others in distress without the buffering that comes from happier interactions. As J. Timothy Davis has remarked, in Tronick's system, an infant engaging with a depressed caregiver will 'learn meanings about self and other that are characterized by depressive affects (helplessness, hopelessness, negativity, etc....) and depressed biology (low serotonin, low energy, etc.)'.[54] It is probably the case that adults living in isolation with other depressed adults will be more likely to form intersubjective systems that have the same negative effects on emotions and biology. This may provide a clue as to why relationally rich environments have such positive impacts on adult, as well as child, health.

It will be apparent that the vision of bioposychosociality that we have sketched out in this chapter is fundamentally rooted in systems biological thinking. Engel's model stressed social belonging but he doesn't seem to have grasped how dynamic the business of meaning-making really is. He was immersed in Bertalanffy's systems theory and in psychoanalysis. Although Bertalanffy himself was sympathetic to psychoanalysis, devoting whole chapters of his magnum opus to it, it is tempting to speculate that Engel never managed to reconcile these two ways of looking at the world in his own mind. Expanding psychoanalytic theories concerning the role of meaning in structuring experience might have enabled him to provide at least the beginnings of an answer to the question of how we transfer information with our environment, which in turn might have unlocked the question of how the organism uses its discretion in respect of the full range of affordances available at any one point in time. What we are describing by way of Tronick, Bruner and others is similar to Maturana and Varela's vision of autopoiesis: a multilevel system of processes of transformation whose unity consists in the preservation of its relational networks.[55]

Our updated reconstruction of how biopsychosocial causation works is consistent not only with developments in biology itself but also in psychology and in the social sciences. Consider by way of example the turn to 4E cognition in psychology. The basic aim of writers working within a 4E perspective is to make representation less central to cognitive science. Traditionally, psychology has portrayed the mind as a machine for representing the world and using its representations to gain purchase over the environment. The world must then be represented as a source of information. Cognition, on this view, is fundamentally about a mind retired from the world applying rules or algorithms to understand what takes place there. 4E cognition opposes this view. It highlights the individual's profound involvement with her surrounding worlds. Those interactions are embodied, embedded, enactive and extended (the four characteristics of 4E cognition). Cognition relies on a body that reckons with the environment, year by year, day by day and even moment by moment. This embodied self is also embedded in a palimpsest of worlds, from the cell through to particular bodily subsystems all the way up to a society and a culture. It is enactive by dint of its bringing about or enacting a world of significance through its embedded embodiment. And it is extended because the environment itself can under certain conditions be recruited as part of the cognitive process, for example when we use a piece of computer software. In this book, we have been concerned not with cognition but with the production of health states and disease states, although the centrality of embodied, embedded, enactive and extended selfhood is no less important for our argument.

4E cognitive psychology also lays great stress on the individual's embodied agency or supported autonomy. It pictures the individual as an active causal power in various spheres; it highlights the role of engagement as a mode of action. The individual perceives his or her environment by engaging with it. Over time, she comes to share in a rich intersubjective life in a variety of personal and social settings. 4E cognition effectively dissolves the disciplinary boundaries separating psychology from second-person neuroscience, from infant research or phenomenology. We think this is the logical terminus for any biopsychosocial theory.

We have striven to make the model of the WEIRD response to illness presented in this book consistent with 4E cognition. Our stress on holding as a way of keeping illness in or out of focus is intended to capture the power of background engagement with intimates, itself a measure of embodied, enactive, embedded and extended modes of knowing. When we mirror someone we model a social world for them. When we 'hold' them we give them a place in that world. The elements of care we described in Chapter Two create a qualitatively new set of affordances which in turn changes the nature of the organism in relation to the environment. The modes of neurobiological synchrony we described in Chapter Three reinforce inclusion. This chapter has sought to bring all these models, derived from so many distinct fields, together.

Conclusion

The WEIRD world has a common-sense, individualistic view of what major illness does to a sick person's life and it runs roughly as follows. Illness is a misfortune but, with the support of family and friends, most people in the rich world do the best they can with it. The person with the illness will be seen by hospital services. They will try to get better. And if full recovery isn't possible, provided they can find it in themselves to do so, they will salvage some of their former life.

We start from a different set of premises. We think that health supports a set of expectations concerning the social world of which most healthy people are barely aware. Major illness shatters these. The person with the illness is seldom in any doubt about this but healthy people often persist in denying the scale of the change. Health is a profoundly normative idea, possibly the most normative idea we have, but, for a variety of reasons, most healthy people fail to see it as such. One way to think about this mismatch is to say they are attached to 'forms of life' (Wittgenstein's term) in which health is taken for granted much of the time. Forms of life, Wittgenstein wrote, are rooted in 'something animal' because man is at bottom 'a primitive being to which one grants instinct but not ratiocination'.[1] They have a foundation in biology that is often experienced consciously and even viscerally. But they are at the same time unique to humans and are always embedded in human culture. It is this instinctual animal and cultural dimension of human life that we have laboured to bring to light in this book, because that is where much of the human response to illness is actually negotiated. This animal and cultural realm – which we could also call psychobiological – is not crude. It is highly sophisticated in its workings. Although it is partly driven by imperatives that are in some sense pre-rational – many of them, we suggest, serving an evolutionary purpose – it is full of creative possibilities. One need think only of the outcomes of mirroring, holding and compassion to grasp something of their creative range. John Dewey famously thought that care was the inevitable outcome of engaging mindfully with something else. Using very different terms, we have made a similar argument in this book. Here is how Dewey puts the matter:

Consider its inclusiveness. [Mind] signifies memory. We are reminded of this and that. Mind also signifies attention. We not only keep things in mind, but we bring mind to bear on our problems and perplexities. Mind also signifies purpose; we have a mind to do this and that. Nor is mind in these operations something purely intellectual. The mother minds her baby; she cares for it with affection. Mind is care in the sense of solicitude, anxiety, as well as of active looking after things that need to be tended; we mind our step, our course of action, emotionally as well as thoughtfully. From giving heed to acts and objects, mind comes also to signify, to obey – as children are told to mind their parents. In short 'to mind' denotes an activity that is intellectual, to *note* something; affectional, as caring and liking, and volitional, practical, acting in a purposive way.[2]

It is pleasing to find that Dewey's prototypical example here is the mother minding her baby.

All of the theories we have drawn upon in this book are rooted in what is now called relational ontology. This entails three things. They all try to explain what it means to be human by considering the many different ways in which humans are constituted in *relationship* with one another. They all see the relations as having a kind of ontological priority over the entities themselves. Our Darwinian commitment to the proposition that humans are group animals designed to live as group animals secures the first point, while the claim that we are different kinds of creatures in the presence of close others secures the second. Finally, the kinds of relatedness with which we are concerned are often not directly cognizable, in real time. They exist in the realm of the taken-for-granted. They are, in short, predicated on different kinds of unconsciousness.

As the medical humanities have come to focus ever more on issues relating to race, class, gender and sexuality, they have become more preoccupied by the big institutional forces shaping illness. These are critically important subjects and their introduction into the field is long overdue. But our intellectual culture as a whole is in danger of losing sight of the importance of unconscious phenomena in human affairs except when considering very specific distortions of thought such as 'unconscious bias'. One of the things we have tried to offer in this book is an account of how several different kinds of unconsciousness come into play in relations between the sick and the healthy.

In their introductory chapter to the *Edinburgh Companion to the Critical Medical Humanities*, Des Fitzgerald and Felicity Callard contrast what they call an integrationist vision of the medical humanities, characterized by attempts to develop a broad understanding of medicine, one that effectively complements biomedicine by placing the latter in a rich multidisciplinary context largely supplied by the humanities, with an 'entangled' approach (their preferred one), distinguished by the effort to bring to light 'sets of as yet undetermined material-semiotic configurations and alignments (bodily, pathological, cultural, human, and so on)'.[3] The integrationist vision, they write, tends to turn the humanities into a kind of 'handmaiden' to clinical practice, while the entangled one opens up ways into 'animacies, vitalities and pathologies, which flow across different practices and preoccupations that then come to be ascribed to the "humanities" and the "biosciences"'.[4] The theory put forward in this book is surely 'entangled' in Fitzgerald and Callard's sense. We are not integrationists in the sense in which they use the term. Our book does, we believe, assemble a previously 'undetermined set of material-semiotic configurations', with the aim of, first, explaining why the relational networks of the sick often thin out so dramatically, and, second, situating this phenomenon in the larger context of humans drawing together and pulling away and the impact these behaviours have on health.

It is nevertheless worth pausing for a moment on that hyphenated term, 'material-semiotic'. OED tells us that the adjective 'semiotic' was for centuries used only in medicine to mean 'Relating to symptoms' (see sense 1). But today, in the wake of Saussure, the most common meaning is OED's sense 3: 'Of or pertaining to semiotics or the use of signs'. The processes we have tried to entangle with one another – normalization in Bartlett's sense of staying in sync with the group; extending or withholding reciprocity in the interaction order; mirroring, holding and compassion; the role of powerful elaborations of coordinated movement, arousal management and meaning-making in developing and intensifying human connectedness; care;

neurobiological synchrony; and so on – all have a material aspect in that they involve doing things with and to the body, with the help of others; and they also have a semiotic aspect in that none of them can occur in the world except through the pursuit and elaboration of signs and *meanings* with those same others. We see our entangled processes as powerful biopsychosocial parameters: constraints (partial ones, to be sure) that determine the potential energy in interactions between people in general and between the sick and the well in particular in WEIRD societies today.

Let us briefly try to distinguish just a few of the different kinds of unconsciousness in play. First, there is the unconsciousness that comes with the struggle for life itself. There is an evolutionary aspect to wanting to stay in sync with the group. Indeed, as we pointed out in Chapter Three, for most of our species' history, it would have been suicidal to want anything else. But there is also the fact that members of WEIRD societies are psychologically oriented and their closest relationships tend to shape what they experience as real. It is the least examined and least conscious aspects of these relationships that are especially significant, according to Winnicott.

With Freud and Kübler-Ross in mind, we might hypothesize that the mere presence of illness inevitably undoes some of the 'generalized social repression' surrounding death.[5] The person with the illness reminds the healthy other of something they are unsure how to address. We are then in the realm of what Norbert Elias, adapting a phrase from Thorstein Veblen, called 'trained incapacity'. It can be awkward for both sides.

We are dealing with a phenomenon distinct from, but with certain resemblances to, tacit racism.[6] There is a comparable background of inequality. As Ivan Illich observed long ago in *Medical Nemesis* (1974), to be diagnosed is to be marginalized:

Diagnosis always intensifies stress, defines incapacity, imposes inactivity, and focuses apprehension on nonrecovery, on uncertainty, and on one's dependence upon future medical findings, all of which amounts to a loss of autonomy for self-definition. It also isolates a person in a special role, separates him from the normal and healthy, and requires submission to the authority of specialized personnel. Once a society organizes for a preventive disease-hunt, it gives epidemic proportions to diagnosis. This ultimate triumph of therapeutic culture turns the independence of the average healthy person into an intolerable form of deviance.[7]

Very often, a financial gap opens up, because the sick person has to give up work. Irrational mistrust creeps in (did Kathlyn Conway eat red meat?). And, not infrequently, misunderstanding hardens into estrangement. It is the difficulty of agreeing, constructing and honouring new expectations that makes it so difficult. How can we even begin that task if it involves making lots of mistakes of which we may subsequently be ashamed?

It is here that the notion of the interaction order described by the microsociologists is so helpful. Microsociology aimed to uncover unspoken systems of meaning attaching to *situations* (not people). Interaction orders are contractual spaces shaped by the expectations generated by the situation in which the interactants find themselves. Some contractual spaces contain more freedom than others because they offer the parties more room for negotiation. But often, the rules of the interaction order become apparent only when they break down. Goffman's colleague and fellow microsociologist Harold Garfinkel thought that there existed a fundamental set of contractual rules that applied to any successful interaction. These revolved around equality and reciprocity. In Chapter Two, we saw many examples of patients looking for signs that their clinicians will find a way to think of them as equals worthy of some sort of reciprocity. Garfinkel called these implicit rules 'Trust Conditions'. Anne Warfield Rawls and Waverly Duck have summarized these as follows: the parties to the interaction must understand the interaction in the same way; their commitment to the rules must be visible; the benefit of the doubt should be given; and each party must affirm the other's observance of the rules and expect to have their observance of them confirmed in turn. It is not hard to see how major illness might violate these basic conditions. By way of illustration, let us put ourselves in the position of one of the people who ran past David and Pauline Rabin in the hotel in San Marino with a hurried 'Hello, David,' with our gaze riveted to the other end of the room. David was not visibly ill at this point but he had made his diagnosis public. Suppose we were to sit down with him – what will he take us to mean by that action? Will he feel obliged to talk about his illness? Will he think we're prying? Will he allow us to control how much we hear about it? With the previously known facts of his life no longer in place, how can we be the same people for one another that we once were? Who will he want us to be *now*? The unspoken systems of meaning underpinning our relationship have changed beyond recognition. It is no doubt for this reason that so many authors of first-person memoirs of major illness have commented that it is one of the peculiar burdens of a diagnosis that the sick person must shoulder most of the social responsibility that it brings in its wake.

It may be appropriate to remark here that the microsociologists' approach to social encounters is based on an assumption that flies directly in the face of received opinion in the WEIRD world. The assumption is this: social reality is constituted from the base up, through ordinary interactions. Within peer groups, the prescribed customs around illness are far less powerful than most people believe. Interactions are made of embodied 'constitutive practices' (to use Goffman's term). They are always 'situated' in interaction orders characterized by witnessable sequential features (greeting someone or introducing them to a third party or taking turns in a conversation). And they are enactive in the sense that they bring forth a situation in which each interactant plays their part. Perhaps the most shocking feature of this theory is the implication that interaction orders can sometimes work against each other in the same society. Rawls and Duck have analysed interactions between Black people and White people in the United States today and found that interactional expectations differ markedly by race. White people routinely qualify or altogether suppress the Trust Conditions in dealing with Black people. 'Black and White Americans', Rawls and Duck write, 'often violate each other's interactional expectations and the resulting judgements of incompetence often have a moral tone.' What makes the matter worse is that Black people are expected to inhabit two distinct interaction orders at the same time. As Rawls and Duck put it, they have to develop what W.E.B. Du Bois in 1897 called 'double consciousness':

> this sense of always looking at one's self through the eyes of others, of measuring one's soul by the tape of a world that looks on in amused contempt and pity. One ever feels his two-ness, – an American, a Negro; two souls, two thoughts, two unreconciled strivings; two warring ideals in one dark body, whose dogged strength alone keeps it from being torn asunder.[8]

We think something similar may apply to the interaction orders inhabited by the sick. The healthy qualify or suppress the Trust Conditions by, for instance, unilaterally and falsely crediting the sick person with all they were once capable of or reducing their capacities to nought. These are drastic responses, even if they are not intended as such. The damage to the agentic self, the confusion it brings about in terms of a pervasive sense of uncertainty about how one is seen by others, results in a spoiled identity for many. And this situation is often aggravated by the constant exposure to healthy people's sunnier life prospects, access to basic recognition and greater financial security. After he published a memoir about recovering from a stroke, the English writer Robert McCrum was surprised to receive hundreds of letters from sick people and their carers describing how illness had cut them off from life as they had previously known it. Many complained they felt under pressure to pretend they were okay. One correspondent wrote: 'There is such a deafening silence about this world of pain, about those people, like us, who have to live their lives in that world, being "brave" as it is called, perhaps putting on an air of "normality", of "happiness" because otherwise it makes others feel too uncomfortable.' McCrum concluded that the chief value of his memoir was that it put him in touch with a group of people he was unaware of until then. 'Severely disabled, or just brushed by the wings of death, these are people living in what I have come to think of as the world of pain.'[9]

The microsociologists describe a world in which humans were highly sensitive to bodily signals as a source of information about the unspoken systems of meaning in the interaction order. A lot can hinge on a question like 'Are they smiling at me or smirking?' or 'Is that person speaking quietly because they're not interested in what I'm saying or is it because they have a condition affecting the voice?' They were aware of the role of the body in interactional dialogue, but they did not theorize it very far. Bodily signals were sources of meaning and as such affected the interaction of which they were a part. But because the microsociologists' overriding concern was with revealing the contract at the heart of any interaction, they paid little attention to the biological impact of exchanges of information. As we have already noted, Goffman at least was less interested in the building up of large-scale understandings over time between individuals because he thought large-scale understandings could unravel very rapidly. There is no very powerful a priori distinction in microsociological work between close and distant others.

It is here that infant research, our next object of entanglement, introduces us to a whole new realm. Infant research is just as invested as microsociology is in the task of uncovering unspoken systems of meaning.[10] But the hypothesis shared by researchers as diverse as Stern, Trevarthen and Beebe is perhaps even more fundamental for our purposes than Garfinkel's Trust Conditions. We are referring here to their conviction that the sensorimotor self orchestrates and subtends every kind of communication that we are capable of. Through bodily activity we project ourselves into the world with the aim of creating shared psychobiological experiences with others. The smooth running of this system has enormous consequences, developmentally, physiologically and psychologically. The unspoken system of meaning uncovered by infant research turns on moments of becoming connected and disconnected physiologically through contact with others.[11] Many of the pioneers of infant research were consciously building on Winnicott's ideas about the developmental function of mothering. The most important difference to register is that we are no longer talking only or even largely about the routinized knowledge of social structures, as we were with the microsociologists, though that is clearly an important part of children's social acculturation. The unspoken system of meanings of the infant researchers is focused more on the relatedness as a dynamic driver of development in its own right. Powerful elaborations of coordinated movement, arousal management and meaning-making *with others* have far-reaching effects on our health. The infant taking an initiative in the company of another person uses the social world to make experience. Intersubjective encounters with other minds are an indispensable precondition for the development of intelligence. The infant researchers showed that emotional systems regulated infant learning and cognitive capacity as well as general physiological well-being. They discovered a range of satisfactions in intersubjective contact unsuspected by the social theorists: emotional, intellectual, biological and developmental. Only a theory of open biological systems can begin to encompass that panoply. Contemporary social neuroscience enables us to understand these effects continuing into adult life in terms of the larger aims our nervous systems are primed to serve. We must feel safe with others if they are to become close which means that the fight–flight reaction of the sympathetic nervous system must be significantly dampened down. Intimates with long histories of feeling safe in one another's presence are more resilient to alterations in circumstances than are non-intimates. This is why the decision to adopt a near or a distant stance vis-à-vis the sick person is so fundamental to our story. The neurobiological background associated with each kind of relationship is completely different. This statement puts infant research at odds with microsociology because it supplies the basis for an a priori distinction between close and distant others.

Winnicott's concept of holding remains a very valuable concept to keep in mind when considering the intimate sphere because it offers a compelling and counterintuitive account of why intimates who are inexperienced with illness are often the last to notice signs of illness in a close other and why those with experience so often have to take it into their own identity. It is the holder's job to make the held person feel omnipotent – beyond the reach of illness – and autonomous. Psychosomatic contagion is a *feature* of being human, not an anomaly, because it enables us to benefit from the strength of the groups to which we belong. The same is true of the containment of unmourned losses and the promotion of transitional experience. These constitute the unconscious system of meanings of holding environments.

The biopsychosocial model envisages the human body as being, among other things, the physiological record of individual life experiences. Bessel van der Kolk tells us in a related but different context that 'the body keeps the score' and that would appear to be the central finding of the Adverse Childhood Experiences studies and most national and international studies of health inequalities.[12] It is social experience that becomes physiologically embedded in the body over the life-course – a 'material-semiotic configuration' if ever there was one – through the stress response, through the workings of the autonomic nervous system, through memory and other higher brain functions and through opportunities for social affiliation.

We have barely mentioned the kind of unconsciousness that most people will be familiar with, namely, the psychoanalytic one. In addition to the projective–introjective traffic that is an integral part of ordinary life, we might also take note of how illness raises long-forgotten personal memories. In a strange and moving memoir, medical anthropologist Todd Meyers describes the interactions he had with a woman of colour he names Beverly (she died in 2008).[13] Beverly was a grandmother who had been recruited as a research subject in a Johns Hopkins study of how people cope with chronic disease. Meyers was assigned to her as a PhD student. Beverly had multiple health conditions: arthritis, migraines, 'dizziness', chronic obstructive pulmonary disease, 'confusion', depression, substance abuse, type 2 diabetes mellitus, hypertension, hepatitis C, obesity, kidney disease, 'voices' and chronic pain. Her living conditions were also precarious. She looked after three grandchildren who had been abandoned by her eldest son, a drug addict. At first, she seemed to Meyers to radiate what Christina Sharpe had characterized as Black Being: 'Black being that continually exceeds all the violence directed at Black life; Black being that exceeds that force.'[14] Before long, Meyers came to realize that Beverly's life could not actually be observed ethnographically, no matter how much time he spent in her company. The chaos and secrecy of her family life, the enormity of the trials that she and her family routinely went through, meant that Meyers became less confident in his ability to see her straight. Beverly and her family also became more interested in tying Meyers up in that chaos and secrecy. Meyers is convinced that on one occasion Beverly attempted to poison him deliberately.[15] On another, one of Beverly's daughters threatened to implicate him in the obscure, brief disappearance of one of Beverly's granddaughters, apparently the victim of abduction and rape (possibly as a way of ensuring his silence about these events). So many aspects of Beverly's situation did not seem to add up. There was no trust in social knowledge of any kind:

> she was many kinds of patients, many Beverlys, scattered across different medical environments; in her house, she was caregiver, and was cared for, frail, and fierce. I was attempting to unify these scattered pieces, these hers, to return them to a single whole that could tolerate the many. My effort may have

been exhaustive – it was certainly exhausting, and very likely annoying from Beverly's point of view, – in the end, there was no wholeness, no repair, no collection of diagnoses to complete a picture – a picture for whom? There were so many pieces, loose pieces of her churning in a sea of other pieces, with a significance that would bob in and out of view.[16]

Beverly's was a very 'unheld' life in Winnicott's sense. At the centre of Meyers' memoir is a long autobiographical sequence in which he recalls a moment in adolescence when he crashed a car he was driving into a tree. The crash was assumed by everyone else to be an accident but it was in fact his suicide attempt. As he drove to Beverly's house this memory would often rise up unbidden from the depths. It was as if he could only meet her life through this memory. Nothing else in his autobiographical experience approached being equal to Beverly and her world.

All of the different kinds of unconsciousness we have just considered – and our list is far from exhaustive – underlie the organism's manipulation of the many different sorts of meanings that shape its relations with its environment. By bringing these to light, we get to glimpse some of the means by which humans exchange information with the environment as well as the consequences for the organism of doing so. These intersubjective, self-regulating and coregulating activities of the organism constitute at least some of the foundations of embodied agency. Understanding their entanglement, we believe, gives us a more accurate picture of what embodied agency actually involves, bringing us closer to the subjective edges of our biopsychosocial nature. These can only be seen in a conceptual space where ontology, epistemology and physiology meet. We have tried to sketch such a space in this book.

We see our endeavour in this book as belonging to a new phase in the medical humanities, one that is preoccupied not so much with critique as with the elaboration of a handful of key concepts that will sustain transdisciplinary dialogue, one that clinical professionals and anyone interested in health from a scholarly point of view will find indispensable. Systems theory offers the best route to such a synthesis in our view. We have stressed the importance of embodied agency. This reflects our immersion in infant research and the biopsychosocial model it illustrates so powerfully. Coming from sociology, Nikolas Rose and Des Fitzgerald have put the emphasis on notions of affordances and ecological niches.[17] What these concepts have in common is that they are all systems-theoretical concepts aiming to capture higher-order phenomena whose effects can be observed at more fundamental levels. The concepts that feature in the first three chapters of this book attempt to deepen our sense of embodied agency. Chapter Four shows why they matter for health over the long term. The philosophy of medicine has long been interested in achieving a synthesis between the phenomenology of embodiment and cognitive science. Perhaps the most successful attempt is the development of 4E cognition. It is this last which has enabled a much broader and deeper transdisciplinary dialogue between philosophy, psychology and physiology than had been possible before. In like fashion, narrative medicine as elaborated by Rita Charon is now measuring and modelling itself against contemporary systems biology. Charon now sees herself as developing systems narrative medicine.[18]

But, of course, emergentism and the systems thinking on which it is based are not new in the medical humanities. Systems thinking was the great hope for the medical humanities in the 1970s. Alan Sheldon, Ervin Laszlo and Howard Brody made important interventions demonstrating its potential for transdisciplinary work involving the humanities, medicine and biology but none had the impact of Engel's early papers.[19] But the epidemiological findings were not available to any of these writers to develop the model. By the 1990s, the field, while retaining its sympathy with systems thinking, became absorbed in the idea of medicine as a set of interlocking symbolic *cultural* systems. One of the many achievements of Arthur W. Frank's book *The Wounded Storyteller* (1995) was that it presented selfhood in illness as an emergent property of how far the sick person remains in command of the totality of their own resources. And Frank was not alone. In a classic article from 1994, Arthur Kleinman and Joan Kleinman lamented how few conceptual tools were available to analyse 'those processes that charter social space and the space of the body (and self) to intersect and interact'. Using post-Cultural Revolution China as their example, they tried to create 'a new object of scholarly inquiry for interdisciplinary research and theory building, one that crosses between the social sciences, the humanities, and psychobiology'. 'In Chinese cultural settings,' they wrote,

> everyday life is configured as a process of social connexions (*guanxi*). These ties with others provide one with moral capital that is literally incorporated into the body as 'face.' Social connections themselves are animated by *renqing* (favor or situated emotion). As a result, networks as well as bodies are energised with *chi* ('vital energy') which is strengthened or weakened, built up or dissipated, made effective or ineffective, owing to the interconnection between the socio moral and the physical (the somatomoral). Both social bodies and human bodies, Chinese traditional theories of health hold, can be vitalized or devitalized, given face or made to

lose face, moralized or demoralized, owing to the sociomatics of social experience.[20]

It would not be hard to translate these claims into the language of contemporary Western epidemiology. Social affiliation supplies a basis for health that is consciously experienced as 'face' – a term traditional Chinese medicine shares with Goffman. Face ramifies into other spheres of endeavour (education, community life, the world of work), which enables social strata to channel good health differentially to different populations. The Kleinmans went on to describe a world in which three paradigmatic symptoms – dizziness, exhaustion and pain – were perceived in early 1980s China as secondary aspects of social experience recorded by the body. This, they argue, is how bodies remembered in post-Cultural Revolution China. We in the WEIRD world lack an understanding as subtle as this. As Michael Marmot points out in *The Health Gap*, most people think that illness is genetic or results from bad behaviour (smoking, drinking, drug taking, poor diet, lack of exercise, promiscuity).[21] These *are* real causes. But the patterns of illness that prevail in the rich West are determined by the biological embedding that comes with social inequality to a much greater extent than is generally understood. As Marmot's collaborator Geoffrey Rose put it: 'The primary determinants of disease are mainly economic and social, and therefore its remedies must also be economic and social. Medicine and politics cannot and should not be kept apart.'[22]

WHAT IS TO BE DONE, more practically? How can we better acquaint the well with the 'world of pain' Robert McCrum stumbled into? We know of course that there are many excellent medical charities and support organizations run by patients and their families. But they form interaction orders of a unique kind. The healthy world is not disturbed by them (and often isn't directly addressed by them). In the first instance, the healthy and the able-bodied need to develop their own version of Du Boisean 'double consciousness' to take account of the social isolation of the ill. There are many ways this can be achieved. The Macmillan Cancer charity's slogan 'A mate with cancer is still a mate' showed how effective a publicity campaign might be. It was a brilliant way of introducing the importance of intersubjective communal life to general notice. Our culture is beholden to the idea that biomedical support is what the sick need more than anything else. But the sick also need authentic contact, as the Macmillan campaign emphasized.

An advertising campaign would be only a first step. Occasionally, diseases come along that create a care-based counterculture that bring the healthy and the sick together. Think of the response of gay men to HIV/AIDS during the 1980s and beyond which we discussed in the Introduction. One of the many beneficial consequences of the buddy system was that it gave people experience of intimate care – something that has become less common today. Or think of the arrangements described in Sandra Butler and Barbara Rosenblum's classic memoir, *Cancer in Two Voices* (1991), which described the lived experience of a gay woman with breast cancer and her partner, helped by a loyal retinue of lesbian activists.[23] It is tempting to conjecture that in these instances membership of an embattled minority was very helpful in bringing the healthy into close contact with the sick. The fact that buddies and feminist activists were each fighting two distinct but overlapping systems of discrimination (the stigma of illness and the stigma of homosexuality) seems to have turbocharged their resolve. Today, to the extent that this counterculture of this sort exists at all in the WEIRD world, it is focused most visibly on mental illness.[24] But it is still isolated indeed. We need groups like these if the healthy are to think creatively about illness.

The public also needs to get to grips with the biopsychosocial nature of human beings. The isolation suffered by the sick and their close others in highly developed societies is especially grotesque given what we now know about the impact of isolation and adversity on human health more generally. By perpetuating it, we deprive ourselves unnecessarily of a morally valuable experience, and throw away the possibility of making use of the findings of the epidemiological, neuroscientific and epigenetic sciences mentioned above in a demographic where their impact is potentially great. We live in a neoliberal world that fetishizes inequality as a condition of social progress. If we want there to be less illness in the world, we need less inequality. And if we want to manage illness better, we need to take stock of what the health sciences are telling us about the impact of social adversity on the body. It is not just a matter of improving healthcare and improving access to healthcare, important though those goals are. It is, more pressingly, a question of improving the ways in which we support *everyone's* autonomy. In the first instance, it means bringing the sick and their close others back in to shared life.

REFERENCES

Introduction

1 Anne Boyer, *The Undying: A Meditation on Modern Illness* (London, 2019), p. 67.
2 S. Lochlann Jain, *Malignant: How Cancer Becomes Us* (London, 2013), p. 46.
3 Rachel Hadas, *Strange Relation: A Memoir of Marriage, Dementia, and Poetry* (Philadelphia, PA, 2011), p. 166.
4 Ibid., p. ix.
5 Albert B. Robillard, *Meaning of a Disability: The Lived Experience of Paralysis* (Philadelphia, PA, 1999), p. 94.
6 Susan Sontag, *Illness as Metaphor and AIDS and Its Metaphors* (Harmondsworth, 2000), p. 8.
7 Adam Mars-Jones's memoir, *Kid Gloves: A Voyage Round My Father* (London, 2015), contains a moving and detailed account of his work in London as a buddy at the very beginning of the AIDS crisis. For a detailed scholarly ethnography of the buddy system, see John MacLachlan, 'Managing AIDS: A Phenomenology of Experiment, Empowerment and Expediency', *Critique of Anthropology*, XII/4 (1992), pp. 433–56.
8 Irving Kenneth Zola, *Missing Pieces: A Chronicle of Living with a Disability* (Philadelphia, PA, 1982), p. 202.
9 Arthur W. Frank, *At the Will of the Body: Reflections on Illness* (Boston, MA, 1991), p. 36.
10 Robert McCrum, *My Year Off: Rediscovering Life after a Stroke*, 2nd edn (London, 2008), pp. xvii–xviii.
11 Joseph Henrich, *The WEIRDest People in the World: How the West Became Psychologically Peculiar and Particularly Prosperous* (London, 2020).
12 See, for instance, William James Earle, 'Critical Review: Some Remarks on Joseph Henrich's *The WEIRDest People in the World: How the West Became Psychologically Peculiar and Particularly Prosperous*', *Philosophical Forum*, LII/3 (2021), pp. 263–72.
13 David Rabin, 'Compounding the Ordeal of ALS – Isolation from my Fellow Physicians', *New England Journal of Medicine*, CCCVII/8 (1982), pp. 506–9.
14 In addition to the works already cited by David Rabin and Robert McCrum,

see also Fergus Shanahan, *The Language of Illness* (Dublin, 2020), especially Chapter 7.

15 See, for instance, Paola Siviero et al., 'Association between Osteoarthritis and Social Isolation: Data from the EPOSA Study', *Journal of the American Geriatric Society*, LXVIII/1 (2020), pp. 87–95, and A. Fuchsia Howard et al., 'Trajectories of Social Isolation in Adult Survivors of Childhood Cancer', *Journal of Cancer Survivorship*, VIII (2014), pp. 80–93. It goes almost without saying that there are hundreds of papers devoted to the social isolation of those with major mental disorders.

16 Erving Goffman, *Stigma: Notes on the Management of Spoiled Identity* (Englewood Cliffs, NJ, 1963).

17 See, for instance, Mark L. Hatzenbuehler, Jo C. Phelan and Bruce G. Link, 'Stigma as a Fundamental Cause of Population Health Inequalities', *American Journal of Public Health*, CIII/5 (2013), pp. 813–21, and the papers in Brenda Major, John F. Dovidio and Bruce G. Link, eds, *The Oxford Handbook of Stigma, Discrimination, and Health* (Oxford, 2018).

18 See, for instance, Candyce H. Kroenke et al., 'Social Networks, Social Support, and Survival after Breast Cancer Diagnosis', *Journal of Clinical Oncology*, XXIV/7 (2006), pp. 1105–11; Feifei Bu, Paola Zaninotto and Daisy Fancourt, 'Longitudinal Associations between Loneliness, Social Isolation and Cardiovascular Events', *Heart*, CVI (2020), pp. 1394–9; Julie Christiansen et al., 'Loneliness, Social Isolation, and Chronic Disease Outcomes', *Annals of Behavioral Medicine*, LV/3 (2021), pp. 203–15; David Cantarero-Prieto, Marta Pascual-Sáez and Carla Blázquez-Fernández, 'Social Isolation and Multiple Chronic Diseases After Age 50: A European Macro-Regional Analysis', *PLoS ONE*, XIII/10 (2018), e0205062. See also many of the papers in Major, Dovidio and Link, eds, *The Oxford Handbook*.

19 A classic contribution is Christian S. Crandall and Dallie Moriarty, 'Physical Illness Stigma and Social Rejection', *British Journal of Social Psychology*, XXXIV/1 (1995), pp. 67–83. But see also Valerie A. Earnshaw, Diane M. Quinn and Crystal L. Park, 'Anticipated Stigma and Quality of Life among People Living with Chronic Illnesses', *Chronic Illness*, VIII/2 (2012), pp. 79–88, and Aisling T. O'Donnell and Andrea E. Habenicht, 'Stigma Is Associated with Illness Self-Concept in Individuals with Concealable Chronic Illnesses', *British Journal of Health Psychology*, XXVII/1 (2022), pp. 136–58.

20 See, for instance, Norbert Elias, *The Loneliness of the Dying* (Oxford, 1985); Atul Gawande, *Being Mortal* (London, 2014); Seamus O'Mahony, *The Way We Die Now* (London, 2016); David Lester, 'The Stigma against Dying and Suicidal Patients: A Replication of Richard Kalish's Study Twenty-Five Years Later', *OMEGA: Journal of Death and Dying*, XXVI/1 (1993), pp. 71–5; Ana Patrizia Hilário, 'The Stigma Experienced by Terminally Ill Patients: Evidence from a Portuguese Ethnographic Study', *Journal of Social Work in End-of-Life and Palliative Care*, XXII/4 (2016), pp. 331–47; Alicia Krikorian,

References

Joaquin T. Limonero and Jorge Maté, 'Suffering and Distress at the End-of-Life', *Psycho-Oncology*, XXI/8 (2012), pp. 799–808; Youngjin Kang, 'Why Are Dying Individuals Stigmatized and Socially Avoided? Psychological Explanations', *Journal of Social Work in End-of-Life and Palliative Care*, XVII/4 (2021), pp. 317–48.

21 The words quoted are from Robert Kurzban and Mark R. Leary, 'Evolutionary Origins of Stigmatization: The Functions of Social Exclusion', *Psychological Bulletin*, CXXVII/2 (2001), pp. 187–208. But see also Megan Oaten, Richard J. Stevenson and Trevor I. Case, 'Disease Avoidance as a Functional Basis for Stigmatization', *Philosophical Transactions of the Royal Society B*, CCCLXVI (2011), pp. 3433–52, and John Tooby and Leda Cosmides, 'Friendship and the Banker's Paradox: Other Pathways to the Evolution of Adaptations for Altruism', *Proceedings of the British Academy*, LXXXVIII (1996), pp. 119–43.

22 Sarah Wendell, 'Unhealthy Disabled: Treating Chronic Illnesses as Disability', *Hypatia*, XVI/4 (2001), pp. 17–33.

23 Bibb Latané and John M. Darley, *The Unresponsive Bystander: Why Doesn't He Help?* (New York, 1970). This was the book that popularized the term 'the bystander effect'.

24 Eric J. Cassell, *The Healer's Art* (New York, 1976, repr. London, 1985), p. 30.

25 Georges Canguilhem, *The Normal and the Pathological*, trans. Carolyn Fawcett and Robert Cohen (New York, 1991), p. 119.

26 Elisabeth Kübler-Ross, *On Death and Dying: What the Dying Have to Teach Doctors, Nurses, Clergy, and Their Own Families* (London, 1969, repr. 1973), p. 18.

27 Ibid., p. 233.

28 The best statement of this theory is in Merleau-Ponty's essay 'The Child's Relation with Others', trans. William Cobb, in Maurice Merleau-Ponty, *The Primacy of Perception and Other Essays on Phenomenological Psychology, the Philosophy of Art, History and Politics* (Evanston, IL, 1964), pp. 96–157.

29 Thomas S. Szasz, 'The Communication of Distress Between Child and Parent', *Medical Psychology*, XXXII/3 (1959), pp. 161–70.

30 Arthur W. Frank, *The Wounded Storyteller: Body, Illness, and Ethics* (London, 1995; revd edn 2013), p. xii.

31 The concept of holding first appears in Winnicott's paper 'Mind and Its Relation to the Psyche-Soma', written in the late 1940s and published in the 1950s. See Lesley Caldwell and Helen Taylor Robinson, eds, *The Collected Works of D. W. Winnicott*, 12 vols (Oxford, 2016), vol. III, pp. 243–56.

32 Dmitri N. Shalin has put forward a brilliant argument to the effect that many of Goffman's preoccupations as a sociologist (stigma, passing, presentation of self) had strong autobiographical roots in Goffman's experiences as a diminutive Jewish Canadian with a wife who suffered from bipolar disorder. He reads Goffman's paper 'The Insanity of Place' as a disguised account of his first marriage. See Dmitri N. Shalin, 'Interfacing Biography, Theory and

221

History: The Case of Erving Goffman', *Symbolic Interaction*, XXXVII/1 (2014), pp. 2–40.
33 Erving Goffman, *Interaction Ritual* (New York, 1967), p. 186.
34 Colwyn Trevarthen, 'Making Sense of Infants Making Sense', *Intellectica*, XXXIV/1 (2002), pp. 161–88, p. 161.
35 For a powerful first-person account of this process, see Denise Riley, *Time Lived Without Its Flow* (London, 2012, repr. 2019).
36 Emmanuel Levinas, 'Substitution', in *Basic Philosophical Writings*, ed. Adriaan Peperzak, Simon Critchley and Robert Bernasconi (Bloomington and Indianapolis, IN, 1996), pp. 79–96, p. 91.
37 Paul Ricoeur, *Oneself as Another*, trans. Kathleen Blamey (London, 1992), p. 192.
38 D. W. Winnicott, 'A Clinical Approach to Family Problems: The Family', in *Collected Works*, vol. V, p. 543.

1 Emergent Illness

1 This idea of trouble as a challenge to the group mind is sometimes traced to the Cambridge psychologist Frederic Bartlett but was developed explicitly by the anthropologist A. Irving Hallowell in the 1950s. See especially his essay 'The Social Function of Anxiety in a Primitive Society' [1941], in *Culture and Experience* (Philadelphia, PA, 1955), pp. 266–76. Hallowell's notion features prominently in the later work of Jerome Bruner, notably *The Culture of Education* (Cambridge, MA, 1996). Its most distinguished exponent in the health humanities today is the cognitive anthropologist Linda C. Garro. See for example her 'Narrating Troubling Experiences' in *Transcultural Psychiatry*, XL/1 (2003), pp. 5–43, and '"Effort after Meaning" in Everyday Life', in *A Companion to Psychological Anthropology: Modernity and Psycho-Cultural Change*, ed. Conerly Casey and Robert B. Edgerton (Oxford, 2007), pp. 48–71.
2 We find versions of this claim in the writings of Wittgenstein and in Spitzer and Endicott's work for the revolutionary revised third edition of the *Diagnostic and Statistical Manual of Psychiatric Disorders*. See Ludwig Wittgenstein, *Philosophical Investigations*, trans. G.E.M. Anscombe, ed. G.E.M. Anscombe and R. Rhees (Oxford, 1953); Robert L Spitzer and Jean Endicott, 'Medical and Mental Disorder: Proposed Definition and Criteria', in *Critical Issues in Psychiatric Diagnosis*, ed. R. L. Spitzer and D. F. Klein (New York, 1978), pp. 15–40.
3 David Mechanic, 'Sociological Dimensions of Illness Behavior', *Social Science and Medicine*, XLI/9 (1995), pp. 1207–16, p. 1208.
4 Populus, *The State of Cancer: Public Attitudes and Beliefs Towards Britain's Biggest Killer* (London, 2018).
5 I. K. Zola, 'Pathways to the Doctor: From Person to Patient', *Social Science and Medicine*, VII/9 (1973), pp. 677–89.

6 Annette Scambler, Graham Scambler and Donald Craig, 'Kinship and Friendship Networks and Women's Demand for Primary Care', *Journal of the Royal College of General Practitioners*, XXXI (1981), pp. 746–50.

7 Blair T. Johnson and Rebecca L. Acabchuk, 'What Are the Keys to a Longer, Happier Life? Answers from Five Decades of Health Psychology Research', *Social Science and Medicine*, CXCVI (2018), pp. 218–26.

8 Susan E. Scott, 'Delay in Seeking Help', in *The Cambridge Handbook of Psychology, Health and Medicine*, ed. Susan Ayers et al. (Cambridge, 2007, repr. 2014), pp. 70–74.

9 Anne Boyer, *The Undying: A Meditation on Modern Illness* (London, 2019), p. 103.

10 Frederic Bartlett, *Remembering: A Study in Experimental and Social Psychology* (Cambridge, 1932).

11 Harvey Sacks, 'On Doing "Being Ordinary"', in *Structures of Social Action*, ed. J. Maxwell Atkinson (Cambridge, 1985), pp. 413–29.

12 Irving Kenneth Zola, *Missing Pieces: A Chronicle of Living with a Disability* (Philadelphia, PA, 1982), p. 227.

13 Ibid., p. 211.

14 Robert McRuer, *Crip Theory: Cultural Signs of Queerness and Disability* (New York, 2006), p. 1.

15 Rosemarie Garland-Thomson, 'The Story of My Work: How I Became Disabled', *Disability Studies Quarterly*, XXXIV/2 (2014), https://dsq-sds.org/article/view/4254.

16 Robert F. Murphy, *The Body Silent: The Different World of the Disabled* (New York, 1987), p. 20.

17 Arthur Kleinman, *The Illness Narratives: Suffering, Healing, and the Human Condition* (New York, 1988), pp. 31–55, p. 48.

18 Bruce G. Link and Jo Phelan, 'Stigma Power', *Social Science and Medicine*, CIII (2014), pp. 24–32.

19 John M. Hull, *On Sight and Insight: A Journey into the World of Blindness* (London, 1997, repr. 2001), pp. 34–5.

20 Eli Clare, *Brilliant Imperfection: Grappling with Cure* (London, 2017), p. 6.

21 Boyer, *The Undying*, p. 170.

22 This scholarship has been brilliantly summarized in Lennard J. Davis, 'Introduction: Normality, Power, and Culture', in *The Disability Studies Reader*, 4th edn, ed. Lennard J. Davis (London, 2013), p. 12. See also Georges Canguilhem, *The Normal and the Pathological*, trans. Carolyn Fawcett in collaboration with Robert S. Cohen (Dordrecht, 1989, repr. New York, 1991); Michel Foucault, *The Birth of the Clinic*, trans. Alan Sheridan Smith (London, 1975); and Ian Hacking, *The Taming of Chance* (Cambridge, 1990, repr. 2013).

23 Hacking, *The Taming of Chance*, p. vii.

24 Zygmunt Bauman, 'Postmodern Adventures of Life and Death', in *Modernity,*

Medicine and Health: Medical Sociology towards 2000, ed. Paul Higgs and Graham Scambler (London, 1998), p. 223.

25 Canguilhem, *The Normal and the Pathological*, p. 186.

26 Michel Foucault, *Discipline and Punish: Birth of the Prison*, trans. Alan Sheridan Smith (London, 1977, repr. 2012), p. 300.

27 Ian Hacking, *Rewriting the Soul: Multiple Personality and the Sciences of Memory* (Chichester, 1995), p. 77.

28 'I think we can see how what I will call "the great maneuvers of hysteria" unfolded at Salpêtrière, and how they were constituted. I will not try to analyze this in terms of the history of hysterics any more than in terms of psychiatric knowledge of hysterics, but rather in terms of battle, confrontation, reciprocal encirclement, of the laying of mirror traps, of investment and counterinvestment, of struggles for control between doctors and hysterics.' See Michel Foucault, *Psychiatric Power: Lectures at the Collège de France, 1973–1974*, ed. A. Davidson, trans. Graham Burchell (Houndmills, 2006), p. 308.

29 See www.gov.uk/reasonable-adjustments-for-disabled-workers, accessed 19 February 2024.

30 Arthur W. Frank, 'Illness and Autobiographical Work: Dialogue as Narrative Destabilization', *Qualitative Sociology*, XXIII/1 (2000), pp. 135–56. The parallel with the experience of gay adults since the 1970s in having to out themselves (and sometime others) to achieve social inclusion is striking.

31 Macmillan Cancer Support, 'A mate with cancer is still a mate', www.youtube.com, accessed 19 February 2024.

32 Frank, 'Illness and Autobiographical Work', p. 137.

33 Ian Hacking, 'Between Michel Foucault and Erving Goffman: Between Discourse in the Abstract and Face-to-Face Interaction', *Economy and Society*, XXXIII/3 (2004), pp. 277–302, p. 292.

34 Sandra Butler and Barbara Rosenblum, *Cancer in Two Voices* (San Francisco, CA, 1991, revd and enlarged 1996).

35 John Bayley, *Iris: A Memoir of Iris Murdoch* (London, 1998), pp. 193–4.

36 Ibid., p. 193.

37 Ibid., p. 194.

38 Sigrid Rausing, *Mayhem: A Memoir* (London, 2017), pp. 39–40.

39 Ibid., p. 38.

40 David Goode, 'Ethnomethodology and Disability Studies: A Reflection on Robillard', *Human Studies*, XXVI/4 (2003), pp. 493–503.

41 Albert B. Robillard, *Meaning of a Disability: The Lived Experience of Paralysis* (Philadelphia, PA, 1999), p. 2.

42 D. W. Winnicott, 'The Theory of the Parent-Infant Relationship', in *The Collected Works of D. W. Winnicott*, ed. Lesley Caldwell and Helen Taylor Robinson, 12 vols (Oxford, 2016), vol. VI, pp. 141–59.

43 Ibid., p. 150.

44 Winnicott, 'The First Year of Life: Modern Views on the Emotional
Development', in *Collected Works*, vol. v, pp. 319–32, p. 319.
45 Winnicott, 'The Theory of the Parent-Infant Relationship', p. 151.
46 Winnicott, 'The First Year of Life', p. 321.
47 Ibid., p. 322.
48 Winnicott, 'The Theory of the Parent-Infant Relationship', p. 151.
49 Ibid., p. 152.
50 Ibid., p. 149.
51 Winnicott, 'The Antisocial Tendency', in *Collected Works*, vol. v, pp. 149–58,
p. 156.
52 Winnicott, 'The Theory of the Parent-Infant Relationship', p. 149.
53 Robert Kegan, *In Over Our Heads: The Mental Demands of Modern Life*
(Cambridge, MA, 1994), p. 43.
54 Winnicott, 'The Theory of the Parent-Infant Relationship', pp. 151–2.
55 Christopher Bollas, *The Shadow of the Object: Psychoanalysis of the Unthought
Known* (London, 1987, repr. 2017), p. 43.
56 Rausing, *Mayhem*, p. 40.
57 Ibid., p. 41.
58 Zygmunt Bauman, *Mortality, Immortality and Other Life Strategies*
(Cambridge, 1992), p. 17.
59 Aristotle, *Nicomachean Ethics*, trans. Christopher Rowe, ed. Sarah Broadie
and Christopher Rowe (Oxford, 2002, repr. 2020).
60 A. W. Price, *Love and Friendship in Plato and Aristotle* (Oxford, 1990), p. 123.
61 Kathlyn Conway, *Ordinary Life: A Memoir of Illness* (New York, 1997), p. 101.
62 Brian Hodges, 'Medical Student Bodies and the Pedagogy of Self-Reflection,
Self-Assessment, and Self-Regulation', *Journal of Curriculum Theorizing*, XX/2
(2004), pp. 41–52.
63 See for example Rachelle A. Dorfman, *Aging Into the 21st Century: The
Exploration of Aspirations and Values* (London, 2013), p. 149.
64 Julia Segal, *The Trouble with Illness: How Illness and Disability Affect
Relationships* (London, 2017), p. 23.
65 Elaine Scarry, *The Body in Pain: The Making and Unmaking of the World*
(Oxford, 1985).
66 Richard Hilbert, 'The Acultural Dimensions of Chronic Pain: Flawed Reality
Construction and the Problem of Meaning', *Social Problems*, XXXI/4 (1984),
pp. 365–78, p. 375.
67 Harold Brodkey, *This Wild Darkness: The Story of My Death* (London, 1996),
p. 96.
68 Dennis Potter, *Seeing the Blossom* (London, 1994), p. 5.
69 Arthur W. Frank, *At the Will of the Body: Reflections on Illness* (Boston, MA,
1991), p. 33.
70 Gillian Rose, *Love's Work* (London, 1994), p. 84. Her other memoir was the
unfinished and posthumously published *Paradiso* (London, 1999).

2 Care

1 Arthur Kleinman, *The Soul of Care: The Moral Education of a Doctor* (London, 2019), p. 101.
2 Hugo Mercier and Dan Sperber, *The Enigma of Reason* (Cambridge, MA, 2017), p. 17.
3 Arthur Kleinman, 'Care: In Search of a Health Agenda', *The Lancet*, CCCLXXXVI/9990 (2015), pp. 240–41, p. 240.
4 Carol Gilligan, *In A Different Voice: Psychological Theory and Women's Development* (Cambridge, MA, 1982, repr. 1993); Nel Noddings, *Caring: A Feminine Approach to Ethics and Moral Education* (Berkeley, CA, 1984); Berenice Fisher and Joan C. Tronto, 'Toward a Feminist Theory of Caring', in *Circles of Care: Work and Identity in Women's Lives*, ed. Emily K. Abel and Margaret Nelson (Albany, NY, 1990), pp. 35–54; Virginia Held, *The Ethics of Care: Personal, Political, and Global* (Oxford, 2006).
5 Their influence can be seen, for instance, in Lisa Baraitser's wonderful book *Enduring Time* (London, 2017), which defines care as 'the arduous temporal practice of maintaining ongoing relations with others and the world' (p. 4).
6 Fisher and Tronto, 'Toward a Feminist Theory of Caring', pp. 35–54.
7 Joan C. Tronto, *Who Cares: How to Reshape a Democratic Politics* (London, 2015), p. 3.
8 Perhaps the most controversial conclusion was that girls were socialized to be morally better than boys.
9 'Carol Gilligan', https://ethicsofcare.org, 21 June 2011.
10 For an excellent overview of this material, see Chapter 3 of Emma Dowling, *The Care Crisis: What Caused It and How Can We End It?* (London, 2021).
11 Arthur Kleinman, 'Presence', *The Lancet*, CCCLXXXIX/10088 (2017), pp. 2466–7.
12 See for example Arlie Russell Hochschild, *The Managed Heart: Commercialization of Human Feeling* (Berkeley, CA, 1983; updated with a new preface 2012); *The Second Shift: Working Families and the Revolution at Home* (London, 1989, repr. 2012); and *The Outsourced Self: Intimate Life in Market Times* (London, 2012).
13 Tronto, *Who Cares*, p. 5.
14 Colwyn Trevarthen, 'Making Sense of Infants Making Sense', *Intellectica*, XXXIV/1 (2002), pp. 161–88, p. 161.
15 Russell Meares, *The Metaphor of Play: Origin and Breakdown of Personal Being*, 3rd edn (Abingdon, 2005), p. 24.
16 Edmund Husserl, *Cartesian Meditations: An Introduction to Phenomenology*, trans. Dorion Cairns (London, 1960), p. 92.
17 The first publication of this group was Vincent J. Felitti et al., 'Relationship of Childhood Abuse and Household Dysfunction to Many of the Leading Causes of Death in Adults: The Adverse Childhood Experiences (ACE)

Study', *American Journal of Preventive Medicine*, XIV/4 (1998), pp. 245–58. Many dozens of publications have followed it.

18 Annemarie Mol, *The Logic of Care: Health and the Problem of Patient Choice* (Abingdon, 2008).

19 Colwyn Trevarthen, '"Stepping Away from the Mirror: Pride and Shame in Adventures of Companionship": Reflections on the Nature and Emotional Needs of Infant Intersubjectivity', in *Attachment and Bonding: A New Synthesis*, ed. C. Sue Carter et al. (London, 2006), pp. 55–84, p. 55.

20 Giannis Kugiumutzakis, Theano Kokkinaki, Maria Makrodimitraki and Elena Vitalaki, 'Emotions in Early Mimesis', in *Emotional Development: Recent Research Advances*, ed. Jacqueline Nadel and Darwin Muir (Oxford, 2004), pp. 161–81; Daniel N. Stern, *Forms of Vitality: Exploring Dynamic Experience in Psychology, the Arts, Psychotherapy, and Development* (Oxford, 2010), pp. 140–41.

21 Meares, *The Metaphor of Play*, p. 24.

22 Husserl, *Cartesian Meditations*, p. 111.

23 Maurice Merleau-Ponty, 'The Child's Relation with Others', trans. William Cobb, in *The Primacy of Perception and Other Essays on Phenomenological Psychology, the Philosophy of Art, History and Politics* (Evanston, IL, 1964), pp. 96–155, p. 118.

24 This point has also been explored in detail by Giuseppe Civitarese in 'Between "Other" and "Other": Merleau-Ponty as a Precursor of the Analytic Field', *Fort Da*, XX/1 (2014), pp. 9–29.

25 This scene is adapted from the first chapter of Beatrice Beebe and Frank Lachmann, *Infant Research and Adult Treatment: Co-Constructing Interactions* (London, 2013).

26 Ernst Bloch, *The Principle of Hope*, trans. Neville Plaice, Stephen Plaice and Paul Knight, 3 vols (Oxford, 1995), vol. III, p. 958.

27 Stern, *Forms of Vitality*.

28 Stephen Malloch and Colwyn Trevarthen, eds, *Communicative Musicality: Exploring the Basis of Human Companionship* (Oxford, 2009), pp. i–xii.

29 Ibid.

30 Colwyn Trevarthen, 'Embodied Human Intersubjectivity: Imaginative Agency, to Share Meaning', *Cognitive Semiotics*, IV/1 (2013), pp. 6–56, p. 11.

31 'Playing on the Right Side of the Brain: An Interview with Allan N. Schore', *American Journal of Play*, IX/2 (2017), pp. 105–42, p. 116.

32 Jay Bernstein, 'Trust: On the Real But Almost Always Unnoticed, Ever-Changing Foundation of Ethical Life', *Metaphilosophy*, XLII/4 (2011), pp. 395–416, p. 413.

33 D. W. Winnicott, 'Playing: A Theoretical Statement', in *The Collected Works of D. W. Winnicott*, ed. Lesley Caldwell and Helen Taylor Robinson, 12 vols (Oxford, 2016), vol. VIII, pp. 299–312.

34 Ibid., p. 307.

35 See, for example, Allan N. Schore, 'The Interpersonal Neurobiology of Inter-subjectivity', *Frontiers in Psychology*, XII (2021), https://doi.org/10.3389/fpsyg.2021.648616.

36 Daniel N. Stern, *The Interpersonal World of the Infant: A View from Psychoanalysis and Developmental Psychology* (New York, 1985, repr. London, 1998), p. 197.

37 Edward Z. Tronick, 'The Increasing Differentiation and Nontransferability of Ways of Being Together', *Journal of Infant, Child, and Adolescent Psychotherapy*, II/4 (2002), pp. 47–60, p. 51.

38 Edward Z. Tronick, *The Neurobehavioral and Social-Emotional Development of Infants and Children* (New York, 2007), p. 369. For a detailed accessible exposition of Prigogine's views see Ilya Prigogine, in collaboration with Isabelle Stengers, *The End of Certainty: Time, Chaos, and the New Laws of Nature* (London, 1997).

39 Harold Garfinkel, *Studies in Ethnomethodology* (Englewood Cliffs, NJ, 1967), p. 36.

40 A version of it appears in his very first published paper, written before he had even begun his graduate studies ('Symbols of Class Status', *British Journal of Sociology*, II/4 (1951), pp. 294–304). The interaction order was also the subject of the last paper he published before his death ('Presidential Address: The Interaction Order', *American Sociological Review*, XLVIII/1 (1983), pp. 1–17).

41 The following account of the interaction order draws heavily on Anne Warfield Rawls, 'Interaction Order *Sui Generis*: Goffman's Contribution to Social Theory', *Sociological Theory*, V/2 (1987), pp. 136–49.

42 The weakness of Goffman's theory is that he does not go beyond mirroring. He was always focused on what transpires in one-off transactions between interactants. He underestimated the role of love and deep knowing on human interactions. He didn't, in other words, distinguish the realm of *philia* from the realm of calculation. For him, there is only calculation.

43 Emile Durkheim, *The Elementary Forms of Religious Life*, trans. Karen E. Fields (New York, 1995).

44 Bernstein, 'Trust', p. 413.

45 Erving Goffman, *Interaction Ritual* (New York, 1967), pp. 84–5.

46 Erving Goffman, *Stigma: Notes on the Management of Spoiled Identity* (Englewood Cliffs, NJ, 1963), p. 2.

47 Erving Goffman, *The Presentation of Self in Everyday Life* (New York, 1959), p. 253.

48 In some respects, this is similar to the psychoanalytic idea that interactions with other people restructure the self. Christopher Bollas holds that encounters with others are inherently traumatic because they bring to an end the sense of self we experienced before the encounter. See Sarah Nettleton, *The Metapsychology of Christopher Bollas: An Introduction* (Abingdon, 2017), p. 44.

49 Colwyn Trevarthen, 'Awareness of Infants: What Do They, and We, Seek?', *Psychoanalytic Inquiry*, XXXV/4 (2015), pp. 395–416, p. 399.

50 Ibid.

51 Hochschild, *The Managed Heart*, p. 4.

52 A version of the trainer's idea can be found in Aristotle's *Nicomachean Ethics*: 'Most people are thought to wish more to be loved than to love, because of love of honour, which is why most people love flattery; for the flatterer is a friend who is inferior, or pretends to be such, and to love more than to be loved, and being loved is thought to be something close to being honoured, which is something most people seek.' See Aristotle, *Nicomachean Ethics*, trans. Christopher Rowe, ed. Sarah Broadie and Christopher Rowe (Oxford, 2002, repr. 2020), pp. 216–17.

53 Albert B. Robillard, *Meaning of a Disability: The Lived Experience of Paralysis* (Philadelphia, PA, 1999), p. 104.

54 John M. Hull, *On Sight and Insight: A Journey into the World of Blindness* (London, 1997, repr. 2001), p. 87.

55 Havi Carel, *Phenomenology of Illness* (Oxford, 2016), p. 118.

56 In fact, a version of this idea can be found in David Hume's *A Treatise of Human Nature* (1739). 'No quality of human nature is more remarkable, both in itself and in its consequences, than that propensity we have to sympathise with others, and to receive by communication their inclinations and sentiments, however different from, or even contrary to our own. This is not only conspicuous in children, who implicitly embrace every opinion propos'd to them; but also in men of the greatest judgment and understanding, who find it very difficult to follow their own reason or inclination, in opposition to that of their friends and daily companions.' See David Hume, *A Treatise of Human Nature*, ed. D. F. Norton and M. J. Norton (Oxford, 2000), p. 208. Hume goes on: 'The minds of all men are similar in their feelings and operations; nor can any one be actuated by any affection, of which all others are not, in some degree, susceptible. As in strings equally wound up, the motion of one communicates itself to the rest; so all the affections readily pass from one person to another, and beget correspondent movements in every human creature' (Ibid., p. 368).

57 Robert F. Murphy, *The Body Silent: The Different World of the Disabled* (New York, 1987), p. 87.

58 Kathlyn Conway, *Ordinary Life: A Memoir of Illness* (New York, 1997, repr. Ann Arbor, MI, 2007), p. 57.

59 Robillard, *Meaning of a Disability*, p. 43.

60 Conway, *Ordinary Life*, pp. 97–8.

61 Robillard, *Meaning of a Disability*, p. 57.

62 David Rabin, 'Compounding the Ordeal of ALS – Isolation from My Fellow Physicians', *New England Journal of Medicine*, CCCVII/8 (1982), pp. 506–9.

63 Irving Kenneth Zola, *Missing Pieces: A Chronicle of Living with a Disability* (Philadelphia, PA, 1982), p. 52.

64 Kleinman has been indefatigable in making this point (for Kleinman, see for example *The Illness Narratives: Suffering, Healing and the Human Condition* (New York, 1988), p. 3, and *The Soul of Care*, pp. 18 and 35, and in numerous articles published between those books); see also Rita Charon, 'Narrative Medicine: A Model for Empathy, Reflection, Profession, and Trust', *JAMA*, CCLXXXVI/15 (2001), pp. 1897–902; Johanna Shapiro, 'Illness Narratives: Reliability, Authenticity and the Empathic Witness', *Medical Humanities*, XXXVII/2 (2011), pp. 68–72. The primacy of witnessing illness more generally can also be found throughout Arthur W. Frank's *The Wounded Storyteller: Body, Illness, and Ethics* (London, 1995; revd edn 2013).

65 Rita Charon, *Narrative Medicine: Honoring the Stories of Illness* (New York, 2006), p. 113.

66 This will be a major preoccupation of Chapter Three.

67 Hélène Mialet, *Hawking Incorporated: Stephen Hawking and the Anthropology of the Knowing Subject* (London, 2012).

68 Desmond O'Neill, 'Protecting Our Second Harvest', *The Lancet*, CCCXCVI/10266 (2020), pp. 1875–6.

69 Paul Ricoeur, *Oneself as Another*, trans. Kathleen Blamey (London, 1992), p. 192.

70 Winnicott, *Collected Works*, vol. IX, p. 194.

71 Neeli M Bendapudi et al., 'Patients' Perspectives on Ideal Physician Behaviors', *Mayo Clinic Proceedings*, LXXXI/3 (2006), pp. 338–44.

72 For an instance of such a clinician, see for example Henry Marsh, *Do No Harm: Stories of Life, Death and Brain Surgery* (London, 2014).

73 Jerome Groopman's *How Doctors Think* (New York, 2007) contains wonderful examples of consultations going awry because of these phenomena.

74 Andrew Lees, 'Words', FitzPatrick Lecture of the Royal College of Physicians of London, 2021, in A. J. Lees, *Brainspotting: Adventures in Neurology* (London, 2022), pp. 79–89.

75 Here he is surely quoting a famous sentence in Michael Balint's classic book, *The Doctor, His Patient and the Illness* (London, 1957): 'the most frequently used drug in general practice was *the doctor himself*, i.e. it was not only the bottle of medicine or the box of pills that mattered, but the way the doctor gave them to his patient – in fact, the whole atmosphere in which the drug was given and taken' (p. 1).

76 For an account of some of the more florid ways in which psychiatric suffering can mimic neurological disorders see Suzanne O'Sullivan, *It's All In Your Head: True Stories of Imaginary Illness* (London, 2016).

77 Royal College of General Practitioners, 'The Power of Relationships: What Is Relationship-Based Care and Why Is It Important?' (June 2021), at www.rcgp.org.uk. The definition of relationship-based care which we have quoted (and which is cited in 'The Power of Relationships') comes from Denis Pereira Gray, George Freeman, Catherine Johns and Martin Rowland, 'Covid 19: A Fork in the Road for General Practice', *BMJ*, CCCLXX (2020), pp. 1–2.

78 Eric J. Cassell, *The Nature of Healing: The Modern Practice of Medicine* (Oxford, 2013), p. xvi.

79 Eric J. Cassell, *Doctoring: The Nature of Primary Care Medicine* (Oxford, 1997), p. 15.

80 This desideratum is the subject of a famous treatise by the physician William Osler, *Aequanimitas* (Philadelphia, PA, 1904). This is an enlarged version of a list given by Winnicott in his paper on 'Cure'. See Winnicott, *Collected Works*, vol. IX, p. 195.

81 Winnicott, 'The Theory of the Parent-Infant Relationship', in *Collected Works,* vol. VI, p. 150.

82 Nicholas A. Christakis and Elizabeth B. Lamont, 'Extent and Determinants of Error in Doctors' Prognoses in Terminally Ill Patients: Prospective Cohort Study', *BMJ*, CCCXX (2000), p. 469.

83 The work of 'Coping with Cancer' is described in Alexi A Wright et al., 'Associations Between End-of-Life Discussions, Patient Mental Health, Medical Care Near Death, and Caregiver Bereavement Adjustment', *Journal of the American Medical Association*, CCC/14 (2008), pp. 1665–73.

84 Sara's case is described in Chapter 6 of Atul Gawande, *Being Mortal: Illness, Medicine and What Matters in the End* (London, 2014), pp. 174–221.

85 Seamus O'Mahony, *The Way We Die Now* (London, 2016), p. 73.

86 Gawande, *Being Mortal*, p. 197.

87 See, for instance, the otherwise excellent chapter 'Breaking Bad News' in Margaret Lloyd, Robert Bor, Lorraine M. Noble and Zack Eleftheriadou, *Clinical Communication Skills For Medicine*, 4th edn (Edinburgh, 2019).

88 Cassell, *Doctoring*, p. 112.

89 Joe Wood, 'Cicely Saunders, "Total Pain" And Emotional Evidence at the End of Life', *Medical Humanities*, XLVII (2022), pp. 411–20.

90 Mol, *The Logic of Care*, p. 8.

91 Ibid., p. 58.

92 Ibid.

93 Ibid., p. 19.

94 Ibid., p. 34.

95 Ibid., p. 11.

96 Ibid., p. 55.

97 Ibid., p. 96.

98 'I have separated out "good care" from messy practices. In real life, good care co-exists with other logics as well as with neglect and errors. Here, I have left out such noise in order to distil a "pure" form out of mixed events' (ibid., p. 10).

99 Annemarie Mol, *The Body Multiple: Ontology in Medical Practice* (London, 2002).

3 The Pariah Syndrome

1 Zygmunt Bauman, *Modernity and the Holocaust* (Cambridge, 1989), p. 192.
2 Anne Elizabeth Moore, 'A Few Things I Have Learned about Illness in America', in *Body Horror: Capitalism, Fear, Misogyny, Jokes* (Chicago, IL, 2017), pp. 45–54, p. 49.
3 David Rabin, 'Compounding the Ordeal of ALS – Isolation from My Fellow Physicians', *New England Journal of Medicine*, CCCVII/8 (1982), pp. 506–9.
4 This anecdote appears in David Rabin and Pauline L. Rabin, 'The Pariah Syndrome: The Social Disease of Chronic Illness', in *To Provide Safe Passage: The Humanistic Aspects of Medicine*, ed. Pauline L. Rabin and David Rabin (New York, 1985), pp. 38–47, see pp. 39–40.
5 Rabin, 'Compounding the Ordeal', p. 508.
6 Ibid., p. 508.
7 Roni Rabin, *Six Parts Love: One Family's Battle with Lou Gehrig's Disease* (New York, 1985), pp. 114–15.
8 Rabin and Rabin, 'The Pariah Syndrome', p. 41.
9 Rabin, *Six Parts Love*, p. 113.
10 Rabin and Rabin, 'The Pariah Syndrome', pp. 44–5.
11 Philippe Ariès, *The Hour of Our Death*, trans. Helen Weaver (London, 1981, repr. 2008).
12 Ernest Campbell Mossner and Ian Simpson Ross, eds, *The Correspondence of Adam Smith* (Oxford, 1987), p. 217.
13 James Boswell, 'An Account of My Last Interview with David Hume, Esq', in *Dialogues Concerning Natural Religion*, ed. Norman Kemp Smith (New York, 1947), p. 78.
14 Stephen W. Porges, *The Polyvagal Theory: Neurophysiological Foundations of Emotion, Attachment, Communication, Self-Regulation* (London, 2011).
15 Rabin and Rabin, 'The Pariah Syndrome', p. 41; Roni Rabin, *Six Parts Love*, p. 156.
16 It is interesting to note that one of the ways in which the Rabins tried to maintain their friendships was by organizing musical soirées. What better way could there be to include David in the rhythmically based dimensions of group life? These initiatives enjoyed mixed success as many of their more musical guests drifted away over time.
17 See for instance, many of the essays in Dacher Keltner, Jason Marsh and Jeremy Adam Smith, eds, *The Compassionate Instinct: The Science of Human Goodness* (London, 2010); Jean Decety and Philip L. Jackson, 'The Functional Architecture of Human Empathy', *Behavioral and Cognitive Neuroscience Reviews*, III/2 (2004), pp. 71–100; Felix Warneken and Michael Tomasello, 'Altruistic Helping in Human Infants and Young Chimpanzees', *Science*, CCCXI/5765 (2006), pp. 1301–2.

18 Charles Darwin, *The Descent of Man* (London, 1871, repr. Princeton, NJ, 1981), p. 82.

19 S. Katherine Nelson-Coffey, Megan M. Fritz, Sonja Lyubomirsky and Steve W. Cole, 'Kindness in the Blood: A Randomized Controlled Trial of the Gene Regulatory Impact of Prosocial Behavior', *Psychoneuroendocrinology*, LXXXI (2017), pp. 8–13.

20 See Julie Lythcott-Haims, *How to Raise an Adult* (New York, 2015). For an excellent popular discussion of 'weathering together' see Bruce D. Perry and Oprah Winfrey, *What Happened to You? Conversations on Trauma, Resilience, and Healing* (London, 2021).

21 This figure is widely cited. We take it from Robert L. Kelly, *The Lifeways of Hunter Gatherers: The Foraging Spectrum* (Cambridge, 2013), p. 167.

22 Writers in this tradition generally use this point to explain some of the dynamics of sexism, racism and prejudice against the disabled. For an excellent summary of its main lines of thought, see Gail Weiss, Ann V. Murphy and Gayle Salamon, eds, *50 Concepts for a Critical Phenomenology* (Evanston, IL, 2020).

23 Iris Marion Young, *On Female Body Experience: 'Throwing Like a Girl' and Other Essays* (Oxford, 2005), p. 43.

24 Bernhard Waldenfels, 'Bodily Experience Between Selfhood and Otherness', *Phenomenology and the Cognitive Sciences*, III (2004), pp. 235–48, p. 239.

25 Charles Sherrington, *The Integrative Action of the Nervous System* (Cambridge, 1906).

26 Waldenfels, 'Bodily Experience Between Selfhood and Otherness', p. 244.

27 Ibid., p. 247.

28 Emmanuel Levinas, *Otherwise than Being; or, Beyond Essence*, trans. Alphonso Lingis (Pittsburgh, PA, 1998), p. 52.

29 Some of the Boston Change Process Study Group's recent work can be found on its website, www.changeprocess.org. The first major publication by the group was Daniel Stern et al., 'Non-Interpretive Mechanisms in Psychoanalytic Therapy: The "Something More" than Interpretation', *International Journal of Psychoanalysis*, LXXIX (1998), pp. 903–21. A special number of the *Infant Mental Health Journal* was devoted to the model. Each member of the group contributed a paper individually to this special number. These papers, along with more recent ones, have been collected in a book, Boston Change Process Study Group, *Change in Psychotherapy: A Unifying Paradigm* (New York, 2010).

30 Boston Change Process Study Group, *Change*, p. 166.

31 See Marilyn A. Austin, Todd C. Riniolo and Stephen W. Porges, 'Borderline Personality Disorder and Emotion Regulation: Insights from the Polyvagal Theory', *Brain and Cognition*, LXV/1 (2007), pp. 69–76; Angela J. Grippo et al., 'Oxytocin Protects Against Negative Behavioral and Autonomic Consequences of Long-Term Social Isolation', *Psychoneuroendocrinology*, XXXIV/10 (2009), pp. 1542–53; and Porges, *The Polyvagal Theory*.

32 Graham Thornicroft et al., 'Evidence for Effective Interventions to Reduce Mental-Health-Related Stigma and Discrimination', *The Lancet*, CCCLXXXVIII/ 10023 (2016), pp. 1123–32.

33 See Pierre Bourdieu, *Outline of a Theory of Practice*, trans. Richard Nice (Cambridge, 1977), p. 72. See also 'Connaissance par le corps' in *Méditations Pascaliennes* (Paris, 2004).

34 Norbert Elias, *The Society of Individuals*, trans. Edmund Jephcott, ed. Michael Schröter (Oxford, 1991, repr. London, 2001).

35 Ibid., p. 181.

36 Ibid., p. 204.

37 Jürgen Habermas, *The Theory of Communicative Action*, trans. Thomas A. McCarthy, 2 vols (Cambridge, MA, 1988); Jean-François Lyotard, *The Postmodern Condition: A Report on Knowledge*, trans. Geoffrey Bennington and Brian Massumi (Manchester, 1984); Zygmunt Bauman, *Liquid Modernity* (Cambridge, 2000); Ulrich Beck, *The Cosmopolitan Vision*, trans. Ciaran Cronin (Cambridge, 2006); David Harvey, *A Brief History of Neoliberalism* (Oxford, 2005); Richard Sennett, *The Corrosion of Character: The Personal Consequences of Work in the New Capitalism* (London, 1999).

38 Ulrich Beck, *Risk Society: Towards a New Modernity*, trans. Mark Ritter (London, 1992), p. 88.

39 Pierre Bourdieu et al., *The Weight of the World: Social Suffering in Contemporary Society*, trans. Priscilla Parkhurst Ferguson, Susan Emanuel, Joe Johnson and Shoggy T. Waryn (London, 2000), pp. 185–6.

40 Ulrich Beck and Elisabeth Beck-Gernsheim, *Individualization: Institution-alized Individualism and Its Social and Political Consequences*, trans. Patrick Camiller (London, 2002), p. 204.

41 Helen Fein, *Accounting for Genocide* (New York, 1979), p. 4. As Zygmunt Bauman has observed, 'The "universe of obligation" designates the outer limits of the social territory inside which moral questions may be asked at all with any sense. On the other side of the boundary, moral precepts do not bind, and moral evaluations are meaningless. To render the humanity of victims invisible, one needs merely to evict them from the universe of obligation' (*Modernity and the Holocaust*, pp. 26–7).

42 Albert B. Robillard, *Meaning of a Disability: The Lived Experience of Paralysis* (Philadelphia, PA, 1999), p. 35.

43 Amelia Karraker and Kenzie Latham, 'In Sickness and in Health? Physical Illness as a Risk Factor for Marital Dissolution in Later Life', *Journal of Health and Social Behavior*, LVI/3 (2015), pp. 420–35.

44 Beck and Beck-Gernsheim, *Individualization*, p. 137.

45 Carlos Dobkin, Amy Finkelstein, Raymond Kluender and Matthew J. Notowidigdo, 'Myth and Measurement – The Case of Medical Bankruptcies', *New England Journal of Medicine*, CCCLXXVIII/12 (2018), pp. 1076–8.

46 Richard Sennett, *Flesh and Stone: The Body and the City in Western Civilization* (London, 1994), p. 18.
47 Ibid.
48 Ibid., p. 33.
49 Ibid., p. 371.
50 Robert Fulton, 'Death and the Self', *Journal of Religion and Health*, III/4 (1965) pp. 359–68, p. 359.
51 Leo Tolstoy, *The Death of Ivan Ilyich*, trans. Hugh Aplin (London, 2013), p. 49.
52 Zygmunt Bauman, *Mortality, Immortality and Other Life Strategies* (London, 1992), p. 17.
53 Sigmund Freud, 'Thoughts for the Times on War and Death', in *The Standard Edition of the Complete Psychological Works of Sigmund Freud*, 24 vols (London, 1953–74), vol. XIV, pp. 273–300.
54 Michel Foucault, *The Birth of Biopolitics: Lectures at the Collège de France, 1978–1979*, trans. Graham Burchell (London, 2008).
55 Arthur Schopenhauer, *The World as Will and Representation*, trans. E.F.J. Payne (New York, 1966), p. 463.
56 Quoted in Joachim Whaley, ed., *Mirrors of Mortality* (London, 1981), p. 1.
57 Theodor W. Adorno, *The Culture Industry*, ed. J. M. Bernstein (London, 1991), p. 109.
58 Ibid., p. 116.
59 Yuval Noah Harari, *Sapiens: A Brief History of Humankind* (London, 2011), p. 412.
60 Robert Kurzban and Mark R. Leary, 'Evolutionary Origins of Stigmatization: The Functions of Social Exclusion', *Psychological Bulletin*, CXXVII/2 (2001), pp. 187–208.
61 John Tooby and Leda Cosmides, 'Friendship and the Banker's Paradox: Other Pathways to the Evolution of Adaptations for Altruism', *Proceedings of the British Academy*, LXXXVIII (1996), pp. 119–43.
62 Ibid., p. 132.
63 Rabin, *Six Parts Love*, p. 156.
64 Richard Lewontin 'Gene, Organism and Environment', in *Evolution from Molecules to Men*, ed. D. S. Bendall (Cambridge, 1983), pp. 273–85, p. 273.
65 Emile Durkheim, *The Rules of Sociological Method,* here quoted in Anthony Giddens's translation, *Émile Durkheim: Selected Writings* (Cambridge, 1972), pp. 64–71.
66 Bauman, *Liquid Modernity*, p. 49.

4 Biopsychosocial Beings

1 George L. Engel, 'The Need for a New Medical Model: A Challenge for Biomedicine', *Science*, CXCVI/4286 (1977), pp. 129–36; and, by the same author,

'The Biopsychosocial Model and the Education of Health Professionals', *Annals of the New York Academy of Sciences*, CCCX (1978), pp. 169–81.

2 For neuroecosociality, see Nikolas Rose and Des Fitzgerald, *The Urban Brain: Mental Health in the Vital City* (Princeton, NJ, 2022); for ecosociality, see Nancy Krieger, 'Epidemiology and the Web of Causation: Has Anyone Seen the Spider?', *Social Science and Medicine*, XXXIX/7 (1994), pp. 887–903, and, by the same author, 'Theories for Social Epidemiology in the 21st Century: An Ecosocial Perspective', *International Journal of Epidemiology*, XXX/4 (2001), pp. 668–77; for biocultures, see the special number of *New Literary History*, XXXVIII/3 (2007), edited by Lennard J. Davis and David B. Morris, devoted to biocultures and containing Davis and Morris's 'Biocultures Manifesto'; for developmental systems theory, see Susan Oyama, Paul E. Griffiths and Russel D. Gray, eds, *Cycles of Contingency: Developmental Systems and Evolution* (London, 2001).

3 Derek Bolton and Grant Gillett, *The Biopsychosocial Model of Health and Disease: New Philosophical and Scientific Developments* (Houndmills, 2019).

4 Engel, 'The Need for a New Medical Model', p. 130.

5 See James J. Gibson, *The Ecological Approach to Visual Perception* (Boston, MA, 1979), pp. 127–8. Arguably a very primitive version of this idea is present in Engel's theory.

6 This is a fundamental principle of systems biological theory and we will explain it in more detail later on in this chapter.

7 The exposome is a term that was coined by the cancer epidemiologist Christopher John Wild in 2005. It comprises 'every exposure to which an individual is subjected from conception to death'. It is made up of three overlapping domains: 'host or endogenous factors' such as 'metabolism, endogenous circulating hormones, body morphology, gut microflora, inflammation, lipid peroxidation, oxidative stress and ageing'; external exposures including 'radiation, infectious agents, chemical contaminants and environmental pollutants, diet, lifestyle factors (e.g. tobacco, alcohol), occupation and medical interventions'; and 'the wider social, economic and psychological influences on the individual, for example: social capital, education, financial status, psychological and mental stress, urban–rural environment and climate'. The second category has been the main focus of epidemiology since the Second World War. The third category encompasses many of what are now called the social determinants of health. Wild has observed that 'different components of the exposome will leave their mark or fingerprint, so that one may travel not only forward from the molecular characteristics to the clinic but also back to the exposures, epidemiology and public health.' Examples of such fingerprints include genomics and proteomics. Because it is designed to map the impacts of biological, psychological and social exposures, the exposome is a thoroughly biopsychosocial idea. See Christopher Paul Wild, 'Complementing the Genome with an "Exposome": The Outstanding Challenge of Environmental

Exposure Measurement in Molecular Epidemiology', *Cancer Epidemiology, Biomarkers and Prevention*, XIV/8 (2005), pp. 1847–50, and, by the same author, 'The Exposome: From Concept to Utility', *International Journal of Epidemiology*, XLI/1 (2012), pp. 24–32.

8 It is a curious feature of Nassir Ghaemi's *The Rise and Fall of the Biopsychosocial Model: Reconciling Art and Science in Psychiatry* (London, 2010) that this author refuses to engage with this idea. Ghaemi confines his attention to the biopsychosocial model in psychiatry but it was always much wider in scope than psychiatry.

9 This notion was developed in the late 1950s. Its authors published a bestselling book about it. See Meyer Friedman and Ray Rosenman, *Type A Behavior and Your Heart* (New York, 1974).

10 Engel, 'The Need for a New Medical Model'.

11 Barry Marshall and J. Robin Warren, 'Unidentified Curved Bacilli in the Stomach of Patients with Gastritis and Peptic Ulceration', *The Lancet*, CCCXXIII/8390 (1984), pp. 1311–15.

12 Susan Levenstein, Steffen Rosenstock, Rikke Kart Jacobsen and Torben Jorgensen, 'Psychological Stress Increases Risk for Peptic Ulcer, Regardless of *Helicobacter pylori* Infection or Use of Nonsteroidal Anti-Inflammatory Drugs', *Clinical Gastroenterology and Hepatology*, XIII/3 (2015), pp. 498–506.

13 Here we draw on David S. Goldstein's *Adrenaline and the Inner World: An Introduction to Scientific Integrative Medicine* (Baltimore, MD, 2006).

14 Selye set out this view in his best-selling book, *The Story of the Adaptation Syndrome* (Montreal, 1952).

15 We owe this biographical information to Theodore M. Brown's chapter 'George Engel and Rochester's Biopsychosocial Tradition: Historical and Developmental Perspectives', in *The Biopsychosocial Approach: Past, Present, and Future*, ed. Richard M. Frankel, Timothy E. Quill and Susan H. McDaniel (Rochester, NY, 2003), pp. 199–218.

16 Accounts of Monica's treatment and wider human development are given in George L. Engel, Franz Reichsman and Milton Viederman, 'Monica: A 25-Year Longitudinal Study of the Consequences of Trauma in Infancy', *Journal of the American Psychoanalytic Association*, XXVII/1 (1979), pp. 107–26. See also George L. Engel, Franz Reichman, Vivian T. Harway and D. Wilson Hess, 'Monica: Infant-Feeding Behavior of a Mother Gastric Fistula-Fed as an Infant: A 30-Year Longitudinal Study of Enduring Effects', in *Parental Influences in Health and Disease*, ed. E. James Anthony and George H. Pollock (Boston, MA, 1985), pp. 29–89.

17 Graeme J. Taylor, 'Mind – Body – Environment: George Engel's Psychoanalytic Approach to Psychosomatic Medicine', *Australian and New Zealand Journal of Psychiatry*, XXXVI/4 (2002), pp. 449–57, p. 451.

18 Bowlby first formulated this theory with James Robertson in an unpublished report in 1965 entitled *Protest, Despair and Detachment*. For an account of

this work, see Robbie Duschinsky's magisterial *Cornerstones of Attachment Research* (Oxford, 2020), esp. pp. 34–6. The theory can be found in vol. III of Bowlby's Attachment trilogy, *Loss, Sadness and Depression* (London, 1980).

19 Engel, 'The Need for a New Medical Model', pp. 131–2.

20 Engel himself was accused of mind-body dualism by Jeffrey P. Bishop. He claims that for Engel, 'Man remains a biological being with the addition of a psychological and sociological overlay' (see 'Rejecting Medical Humanism: Medical Humanities and the Metaphysics of Medicine', *Journal of Medical Humanities*, XXIX (2008), pp. 15–25, p. 15). We hope our discussion will show that this view is misguided.

21 David Rosenthal, 'A Suggested Conceptual Framework', in *The Genain Quadruplets: A Case Study and Theoretical Analysis of Heredity and Environment in Schizophrenia*, ed. David Rosenthal (New York, 1963), pp. 505–11.

22 The Danish–American Schizophrenia Study has been criticized for using the notion of a 'schizophrenic spectrum', a more capacious category than the DSM criteria for schizophrenia then in use. If Kety had used the DSM criteria, he would have found no difference between the case and the control group. See Jay Joseph, 'The Danish-American Adoptees Family Studies of Kety and Associates: Do They Provide Evidence in Support of the Genetic Basis of Schizophrenia?', *Genetic, Social, and General Psychology Monographs*, CXXVII/3 (2001), pp. 241–78.

23 Seymour S. Kety, 'From Rationalisation to Reason', *American Journal of Psychiatry*, CXXXI/9 (1974), pp. 957–63.

24 Bertalanffy introduced the idea in 'The Theory of Open Systems in Physics and Biology', *Science*, CXI/2872 (1950), pp. 23–9, and expanded on it at length in Ludwig von Bertalanffy, *General Systems Theory: Foundations, Development, Applications* (New York, 1968).

25 Ilya Prigogine and Isabelle Stengers, *Order Out of Chaos: Man's New Dialogue with Nature* (London, 1984).

26 Alon Lab, 'Systems Biology Course 2018 Uri Alon – Lecture 1 – Basic Concepts', www.youtube.com, 13 May 2018. See also Uri Alon, *An Introduction to Systems Biology: Design Principles of Biological Circuits* (London, 2013, revd 2nd edn 2020), pp. 1–3.

27 Robert M. Sapolsky, *Behave: The Biology of Humans at Our Best and Worst* (London, 2018), p. 236; emphasis in original.

28 Bolton and Gillett, *The Biopsychosocial Model of Health and Disease*, p. 97. The idea of free spaces is intended to capture the fact that there are combinatorial possibilities which create space for molecular diversity and, as a result, for different states of the same organism. Free spaces are thus distinct from affordances.

29 The background to Whitehall I is described in Michael Marmot and Eric Bruner, 'Cohort Profile: The Whitehall II Study', *International Journal of Epidemiology*, XXXIV/2 (2005), pp. 251–6, especially pp. 251–2.

30 Geoffrey Rose, 'Strategy of Prevention: Lessons from Cardiovascular Disease', *BMJ*, CCLXXXII (1981), pp. 1847–51.

31 Michael Marmot, Martin Shipley and Geoffrey Rose, 'Inequalities in Death – Specific Explanations of a General Pattern?', *The Lancet*, CCCXXIII/8384 (1984), pp. 1003–6.

32 Marmot and Brunner, 'Cohort Profile', p. 252.

33 Michael Marmot et al., 'Health Inequalities Among British Civil Servants: The Whitehall II Study', *The Lancet*, CCCXXXVII/8754 (1991), pp. 1387–93.

34 Stephen Stansfeld, Rebecca Fuhrer, Martin Shipley and Michael Marmot, 'Work Characteristics Predict Psychiatric Disorder: Prospective Results from the Whitehall II Study', *Occupational and Environmental Medicine*, LVI/5 (1999), pp. 302–7.

35 Stephen Stansfeld et al., 'Social Inequalities in Depressive Symptoms and Physical Functioning in the Whitehall II Study: Exploring a Common Cause Explanation', *Journal of Epidemiology and Community Health*, LVII/5 (2003), pp. 361–7.

36 It has been replicated and enlarged by similar studies in Finland and Japan. A 'Whitehall in Washington' study has been discussed by the National Institutes of Health.

37 These figures are taken from Michael Marmot et al., *Health Equity in England: The Marmot Review 10 Years On* (London, 2020), pp. 14–18.

38 Marmot addressed this question in his book, *Status Syndrome: How Your Place on the Social Gradient Directly Affects Your Health* (London, 2004, revd 2015).

39 Commission on the Social Determinants of Health, *Closing the Gap in a Generation: Health Equity through Action on the Social Determinants of Health* (Geneva, 2008), p. 1.

40 An excellent summary of this literature can be found in Robert M. Sapolsky, *Why Zebras Don't Get Ulcers* (London, 1998, revd 2004).

41 This material derives from Sapolsky's *Why Zebras Don't Get Ulcers*. Selye didn't understand the primary role of the hypothalamus in triggering the stress response.

42 Vincent J. Felitti et al., 'Relationship of Childhood Abuse and Household Dysfunction to Many of the Leading Causes of Death in Adults: The Adverse Childhood Experiences (ACE) Study', *American Journal of Preventive Medicine*, XIV/4 (1998), pp. 245–8.

43 Erin Hambrick, Thomas W. Brawner and Bruce D. Perry, 'Timing of Early-Life Stress and the Development of Brain-Related Capacities', *Frontiers in Behavioral Neuroscience*, 6 August 2019, https://doi.org/10.3389/fnbeh.2019.00183.

44 Jay Belsky, Avshalom Caspi, Terrie E. Moffitt and Richie Poulton, *The Origins of You: How Childhood Shapes Later Life* (London, 2020), p. 333.

45 Robert F. Anda et al., 'The Enduring Effects of Abuse and Related Adverse Experiences in Childhood: A Convergence of Evidence from Neurobiology

and Epidemiology', *European Archives of Psychiatry and Clinical Neuroscience*, CCLVI/3 (2006), pp. 174–86.

46 M. Champoux et al., 'Serotonin Transporter Gene Polymorphism, Differential Early Rearing, and Behavior in Rhesus Monkey Neonates', *Molecular Psychiatry*, VII (2002), pp. 1058–63.

47 Belsky et al., *The Origins of You*, pp. 291–7.

48 Some of this work is presented in John T. Cacioppo, Stephanie Cacioppo, John P. Capitanio and Steven W. Cole, 'The Neuroendocrinology of Social Isolation', *Annual Review of Psychology*, LXVI (2015), pp. 733–67. See also Cacioppo's earlier book on loneliness jointly written with William Patrick, *Loneliness: Human Nature and the Need for Social Connection* (London, 2008).

49 Amartya Sen, *Inequality Reexamined* (Oxford, 1992).

50 Jerome Bruner, *Acts of Meaning* (London, 1990), especially Chapter 4.

51 Ibid., p. 52.

52 Edward Z. Tronick, *The Neurobehavioral and Social-Emotional Development of Infants and Children* (London, 2007), p. 2.

53 Edward Z. Tronick, 'Why Is Connection with Others So Critical? The Formation of Dyadic States of Consciousness and the Expansion of Individuals' States of Consciousness: Coherence Governed Selection and the Co-Creation of Meaning Out of Messy Meaning Making', in *Emotional Development: Recent Research Advances*, ed. Jacqueline Nadel and David Muir (New York, 2005), pp. 293–315.

54 J. Timothy Davis, 'Even More Than the "Something More": Tronick's Dyadic Expansion of Consciousness Model and the Expansion of Child Psychoanalytic Technique', *Psychoanalytic Inquiry*, XXXV/4 (2015), pp. 430–44, pp. 433–4.

55 Humberto R. Maturana and Francisco Varela, *Autopoeisis and Cognition: The Realization of the Living* (London, 1980).

Conclusion

1 Ludwig Wittgenstein, *On Certainty*, trans. Denis Paul and G.E.M. Anscombe, ed. G.E.M. Anscombe and G. H. von Wright (Oxford, 1975), p. 62.

2 John Dewey, *Art as Experience* (New York, 1980), p. 263.

3 Des Fitzgerald and Felicity Callard, 'Entangling the Medical Humanities', in *The Edinburgh Companion to the Critical Medical Humanities*, ed. Anne Whitehead and Angela Woods (Edinburgh, 2016), pp. 35–49, p. 41. Fitzgerald and Callard explicitly draw inspiration from the work of Karen Barad, a philosopher of physics interested in the foundations of quantum physics. See Karen Barad, *Meeting the Universe Halfway: Quantum Physics and the Entanglement of Matter and Meaning* (Durham, NC, 2006).

4 Fitgerald and Callard, 'Entangling the Medical Humanities'.

5 The phrase is Kübler-Ross's. When Kathlyn Conway told her friends she had breast cancer, she often felt she was letting them down by reminding them of other friends or relatives who had died. See Kathlyn Conway, *Ordinary Life: A Memoir of Illness* (New York, 1997, repr. Ann Arbor, MI, 2007), p. 82.

6 Here we wish to acknowledge the inspirational role of Anne Warfield Rawls and Waverly Duck's book, *Tacit Racism* (London, 2020). These authors point out that many currently popular ways of thinking about tacit racism reduce the problem to *racists* rather than *racism*. Thinking about racism in terms of 'micro-aggressions' or 'implicit bias', they argue, locates the problem in only one party to the interaction. As ethnomethodologists, Rawls and Duck treat interactional expectations themselves as 'structures of racism' that then get institutionalized at the level of ordinary social interaction in ways that often go unnoticed. We think something similar occurs with major illness. Interactional expectations between the well and the ill do not always amount to 'structures of physical health stigma', but because the trust conditions underpinning the relationship are often subjected to comprehensive transformation by the illness process, both sides can be wrong-footed in ways that are hard to articulate in real time.

7 Ivan Illich, *Limits to Medicine: Medical Nemesis: The Expropriation of Health* (London, 1974, revd edn 1995, repr. 2001), pp. 100–101.

8 W.E.B. Du Bois, 'The Strivings of the Negro People' [1897], in *The Souls of Black Folk* (Boston, MA, 1997), p. 38.

9 Robert McCrum, *My Year Off: Rediscovering Life after a Stroke*, 2nd edn (London, 2008), p. xix.

10 Given the etymology of the word 'infant' – the Latin *infans* means 'unable to speak' – perhaps this should not surprise us.

11 It is this model that the Boston Change Process Study Group has tried to use as the prototype for adult psychotherapy. Significantly, a split occurred in the group over how far the power to change lies in the child's autonomously *choosing* to make connections (the majority position) or how far it actually depends on the dyad's capacity to repair misalignments (the minority position represented by Edward Z. Tronick and Alexandra Harrison). See Edward Z. Tronick, *The Neurobehavioral and Social-Emotional Development of Infants and Children* (London, 2007), p. 14.

12 Bessel van der Kolk, *The Body Keeps the Score: Brain, Mind and Body in the Healing of Trauma* (London, 2014).

13 Todd Meyers, *All That Was Not Her* (London, 2022).

14 Ibid., p. 8.

15 Ibid., p. 161.

16 Ibid., pp. 49–50.

17 Nikolas Rose and Des Fitzgerald, *The Urban Brain: Mental Health in the Vital City* (Princeton, NJ, 2022), pp. 188–91.

18 See her entry on 'Narrative Medicine' in *The Palgrave Encyclopaedia of the Health Humanities*, ed. Paul Crawford and Paul Kadetz (Houndsmills, 2020).

19 Alan Sheldon, 'Toward a General Theory of Disease and Medical Care', in *Systems and Medical Care*, ed. Alan Sheldon, Frank Baker and Curtis P. McLaughlin (Cambridge, MA, 1970), pp. 84–125; Ervin Laszlo, *The Systems View of the World* (New York, 1972); and Howard Brody, 'The Systems View of Man: Implications for Medicine, Science, and Ethics', *Perspectives in Biology and Medicine*, XVII/1 (1973), pp. 71–92.

20 Arthur Kleinman and Joan Kleinman, 'How Bodies Remember: Social Memory and Bodily Experience of Criticism, Resistance, and Delegitimation following China's Cultural Revolution', *New Literary History*, XXV/3 (1994) (Part 1), pp. 707–23. Similar paradigms have been outlined in relation to other cultures, notably by Didier Fassin in *When Bodies Remember: Experiences and Politics of Aids in South Africa*, trans. Amy Jacobs and Gabrielle Varro (London, 2007).

21 Michael Marmot, *The Health Gap: The Challenge of an Unequal World* (London, 2015), pp. 9–10.

22 Geoffrey Arthur Rose, *Rose's Strategy of Preventive Medicine* (Oxford, 1992, repr. 2008), p. 161.

23 Sandra Butler and Barbara Rosenblum, *Cancer in Two Voices* (San Francisco, CA, 1991, revd and enlarged 1996).

24 The campaign in the USA against the Sackler family as the owners of the manufacturer and marketer of OxyContin is perhaps another example.

BIBLIOGRAPHY

Ariès, Philippe, *The Hour of Our Death*, trans. Helen Weaver (London, 1981, repr. 2008)

Balint, Michael, *The Doctor, His Patient and the Illness* (London, 1957)

Baraitser, Lisa, *Enduring Time* (London, 2017)

Bartlett, Frederic, *Remembering: A Study in Experimental and Social Psychology* (Cambridge, 1932)

Bauman, Zygmunt, *Modernity and the Holocaust* (Cambridge, 1989)

——, *Mortality, Immortality and Other Life Strategies* (Cambridge, 1992)

Bayley, John, *Iris: A Memoir of Iris Murdoch* (London, 1998)

Beck, Ulrich, *The Cosmopolitan Vision*, trans. Ciaran Cronin (Cambridge, 2006)

——, *Risk Society: Towards a New Modernity*, trans. Mark Ritter (London, 1992)

Belsky, Jay, Avshalom Caspi, Terrie E. Moffitt and Richie Poulton, *The Origins of You: How Childhood Shapes Later Life* (London, 2020)

Bertalanffy, Ludwig von, *General Systems Theory: Foundations, Development, Applications* (New York, 1968)

Bollas, Christopher, *The Shadow of the Object: Psychoanalysis of the Unthought Known* (London, 1987, repr. 2017)

Bolton, Derek, and Grant Gillett, *The Biopsychosocial Model of Health and Disease: New Philosophical and Scientific Developments* (Houndmills, 2019)

Boston Change Process Study Group, *Change in Psychotherapy: A Unifying Paradigm* (New York, 2010)

Bourdieu, Pierre, *Outline of a Theory of Practice*, trans. Richard Nice (Cambridge, 1977)

——, et al., *The Weight of the World: Social Suffering in Contemporary Society*, trans. Priscilla Parkhurst Ferguson, Susan Emanuel, Joe Johnson and Shoggy T. Waryn (London, 2000)

Boyer, Anne, *The Undying: A Meditation on Modern Illness* (London, 2019)

Bruner, Jerome, *Acts of Meaning* (London, 2000)

Butler, Sandra, and Barbara Rosenblum, *Cancer in Two Voices* (San Francisco, CA, 1991, revd and enlarged 1996)

Caldwell, Lesley, and Helen Taylor Robinson, eds, *The Collected Works of D. W. Winnicott*, 12 volumes (Oxford, 2016)

Canguilhem, Georges, *The Normal and the Pathological*, trans. Carolyn Fawcett and Robert Cohen (Dordrecht, 1989, repr. New York, 1991)

Carel, Havi, *Phenomenology of Illness* (Oxford, 2016)

Cassell, Eric J., *Doctoring: The Nature of Primary Care Medicine* (Oxford, 1997)

——, *The Healer's Art* (New York, 1976, repr. London, 1985)

——, *The Nature of Healing: The Modern Practice of Medicine* (Oxford, 2013)

Charon, Rita, *Narrative Medicine: Honoring the Stories of Illness* (New York, 2006)

Clare, Eli, *Brilliant Imperfection: Grappling With Cure* (London, 2017)

Commission on the Social Determinants of Health, *Closing the Gap in a Generation: Health Equity through Action on the Social Determinants of Health* (Geneva, 2008)

Conway, Kathlyn, *Ordinary Life: A Memoir of Illness* (New York, 1997, repr. Ann Arbor, MI, 2007)

Crandall, Christian S., and Dallie Moriarty, 'Physical Illness Stigma and Social Rejection', *British Journal of Social Psychology*, XXXIV/1 (1995), pp. 67–83

Darwin, Charles, *The Descent of Man* (London, 1871, repr. Princeton, NJ, 1981)

Davis, Lennard J., ed., *The Disability Studies Reader*, 4th edn (London, 2013)

Dewey, John, *Art as Experience* (New York, 1980)

Dowling, Emma, *The Care Crisis: What Caused It and How Can We End It?* (London, 2021)

Duchinsky, Robbie, *Cornerstones of Attachment Research* (Oxford, 2020)

Durkheim, Emile, *The Elementary Forms of Religious Life*, trans. Karen E. Fields (New York, 1995)

Earle, William James, 'Critical Review: Some Remarks on Joseph Henrich's *The WEIRDest People in the World. How the West Became Psychologically Peculiar and Particularly Prosperous*', *Philosophical Forum*, LII/3 (2021), pp. 263–72

Earnshaw, Valerie A., Diane M. Quinn and Crystal L. Park, 'Anticipated Stigma and Quality of Life among People Living with Chronic Illnesses', *Chronic Illness*, VIII/2 (2012), pp. 79–88

Elias, Norbert, *The Loneliness of the Dying* (Oxford, 1985)

——, *The Society of Individuals*, trans. Edmund Jephcott, ed. Michael Schröter (Oxford, 1991, repr. London, 2001)

Engel, George L., 'The Need for a New Medical Model: A Challenge for Biomedicine', *Science*, CXCVI/4286 (1977), pp. 129–36

Fein, Helen, *Accounting for Genocide* (New York, 1979)

Fisher, Berenice, and Joan C. Tronto, 'Toward a Feminist Theory of Caring', in *Circles of Care: Work and Identity in Women's Lives*, ed. Emily K. Abel and Margaret Nelson (Albany, NY, 1990), pp. 36–54

Foucault, Michel, *The Birth of Biopolitics: Lectures at the Collège de France, 1978–1979*, trans. Graham Burchell (London, 2008)

——, *The Birth of the Clinic*, trans. Alan Sheridan Smith (London, 1975)

——, *Discipline and Punish: Birth of the Prison*, trans. Alan Sheridan Smith (London, 1977, repr. 2012)

Frank, Arthur W., *At the Will of the Body: Reflections on Illness* (Boston, MA, 1991)

——, *The Wounded Storyteller: Body, Illness, and Ethics* (London, 1995; revd edn 2013)

Freud, Sigmund, 'Thoughts for the Times on War and Death', in *The Standard Edition of the Complete Psychological Works of Sigmund Freud*, 24 vols (London, 1953–74), vol. XIV, pp. 273–300

Garfinkel, Harold, *Studies in Ethnomethodology* (Englewood Cliffs, NJ, 1967)

Garland-Thomson, Rosemarie, 'The Story of My Work: How I Became Disabled', *Disability Studies Quarterly*, XXXIV/2 (2014), https://dsq-sds.org/article/view/4254

Gawande, Atul, *Being Mortal: Illness, Medicine and What Matters in the End* (London, 2014)

Gilligan, Carol, *In a Different Voice: Psychological Theory and Women's Development* (Cambridge, MA, 1982, repr. 1993)

Goffman, Erving, *Interaction Ritual* (New York, 1967)

——, *The Presentation of Self in Everyday Life* (New York, 1959)

——, *Stigma: Notes on the Management of Spoiled Identity* (Englewood Cliffs, NJ, 1963)

Goldstein, David, *Adrenaline and the Inner World: An Introduction to Scientific Integrative Medicine* (Baltimore, MD, 2006)

Goode, David, 'Ethnomethodology and Disability Studies: A Reflection on Robillard', *Human Studies*, XXVI/4 (2003), pp. 493–503

Hacking, Ian, *The Taming of Chance* (Cambridge, 1990, repr. 2013)

Hadas, Rachel, *Strange Relation: A Memoir of Marriage, Dementia, and Poetry* (Philadelphia, PA, 2011)

Hallowell, Arthur Irving, *Culture and Experience* (Philadelphia, PA, 1955)

Hatzenbuehler, Mark L., Jo C. Phelan and Bruce G. Link, 'Stigma as a Fundamental Cause of Population Health Inequalities', *American Journal of Public Health*, CIII/5 (2013), pp. 813–21

Heaney, Seamus, *Human Chain* (London, 2010)

Henrich, Joseph, *The WEIRDest People in the World: How the West Became Psychologically Peculiar and Particularly Prosperous* (London, 2020)

Hilário, Ana Patrizia, 'The Stigma Experienced by Terminally Ill Patients: Evidence from a Portuguese Ethnographic Study', *Journal of Social Work in End-of-Life and Palliative Care*, XII/4 (2016), pp. 331–47

Hochschild, Arlie Russell, *The Managed Heart: Commercialization of Human Feeling* (Berkeley, CA, 2012)

——, *The Outsourced Self: Intimate Life in Market Times* (London, 2012)

——, *The Second Shift: Working Families and the Revolution at Home* (London, 1989, repr. 2012)

Hull, John M., *On Sight and Insight: A Journey into the World of Blindness* (London 1997, repr. 2001)

Hume, David, *A Treatise of Human Nature*, ed. D. F. Norton and M. J. Norton (Oxford, 2000)

Husserl, Edmund, *Cartesian Meditations: An Introduction to Phenomenology*, trans. Dorion Cairns (London, 1960)

Illich, Ivan, *Limits to Medicine: Medical Nemesis: The Expropriation of Health* (London, 1974, revd edn 1995, repr. 2001)

Jain, S. Lochlann, *Malignant: How Cancer Becomes Us* (London, 2018)

Kegan, Robert, *In Over Our Heads: The Mental Demands of Modern Life* (Cambridge, MA, 1994)

Keltner, Dacher, Jason Marsh and Jeremy Adam Smith, eds, *The Compassionate Instinct: The Science of Human Goodness* (London, 2010)

Kleinman, Arthur, *The Illness Narratives: Suffering, Healing, and the Human Condition* (New York, 1988)

—, *The Soul of Care: The Moral Education of a Doctor* (London, 2019)

Kübler-Ross, Elisabeth, *On Death and Dying: What the Dying Have to Teach Doctors, Nurses, Clergy, and Their Own Families* (London, 1969, repr. 1973)

Kurzban, Robert, and Mark R. Leary, 'Evolutionary Origins of Stigmatization: The Functions of Social Exclusion', *Psychological Bulletin*, CXXVII/2 (2001), pp. 187–208

Latané, Bibb, and John M. Darley, *The Unresponsive Bystander: Why Doesn't He Help?* (New York, 1970)

Lees, Andrew J., *Brainspotting: Adventures in Neurology* (London, 2022)

Lester, David, 'The Stigma against Dying and Suicidal Patients: A Replication of Richard Kalish's Study Twenty-Five Years Later', *OMEGA: Journal of Death and Dying*, XXVI/1 (1993), pp. 71–5

Levinas, Emmanuel, *Otherwise than Being; or, Beyond Essence*, trans. Alphonso Lingis (Pittsburgh, PA, 1998)

McCrum, Robert, *My Year Off: Rediscovering Life After a Stroke*, 2nd edn (London, 2008)

MacLachlan, John, 'Managing AIDS: A Phenomenology of Experiment, Empowerment and Expediency', *Critique of Anthropology*, XII/4 (1992), pp. 433–56

McRuer, Robert, *Crip Theory: Cultural Signs of Queerness and Disability* (New York, 2006)

Major, Brenda, John F. Dovidio and Bruce G. Link, eds, *The Oxford Handbook of Stigma, Discrimination, and Health* (Oxford, 2018)

Malloch, Stephen, and Colwyn Trevarthen, eds, *Communicative Musicality: Exploring the Basis of Human Companionship* (Oxford, 2009)

Marmot, Michael, *The Health Gap: The Challenge of an Unequal World* (London, 2015)

—, *Status Syndrome: How Your Place on the Social Gradient Directly Affects Your Health* (London, 2004, revd 2015)

Mars-Jones, Adam, *Kid Gloves: A Voyage Round My Father* (London, 2015)

Meares, Russell, *The Metaphor of Play: Origin and Breakdown of Personal Being*, 3rd edn (Abingdon, 2005)

Mercier, Hugo, and Dan Sperber, *The Enigma of Reason* (Cambridge, MA, 2017)

Merleau-Ponty, Maurice, *The Primacy of Perception and Other Essays on Phenomenological Psychology, the Philosophy of Art, History and Politics* (Evanston, IL, 1964)

Meyers, Todd, *All That Was Not Her* (London, 2022)

Mialet, Hélène, *Hawking Incorporated: Stephen Hawking and the Anthropology of the Knowing Subject* (London, 2012)

Mol, Annemarie, *The Body Multiple: Ontology in Medical Practice* (London, 2002)

——, *The Logic of Care: Health and the Problem of Patient Choice* (Abingdon, 2008)

Moore, Anne Elizabeth, *Body Horror: Capitalism, Fear, Misogyny, Jokes* (Chicago, IL, 2017)

Murphy, Robert F., *The Body Silent: The Different World of the Disabled* (New York, 1987)

Nettleton, Sarah, *The Metapsychology of Christopher Bollas: An Introduction* (Abingdon, 2017)

Oaten, Megan, Richard J. Stevenson and Trevor I. Case, 'Disease Avoidance as a Functional Basis for Stigmatization', *Philosophical Transactions of the Royal Society B*, CCCLXVI (2011), pp. 3433–52

O'Donnell, Aisling T., and Andrea E. Habenicht, 'Stigma Is Associated with Illness Self-Concept in Individuals with Concealable Chronic Illnesses', *British Journal of Health Psychology*, XXVII/1 (2022), pp. 136–58

O'Mahony, Seamus, *The Way We Die Now* (London, 2016)

O'Neill, Desmond, 'Protecting Our Second Harvest', *The Lancet*, CCCXCVI/10266 (2020), pp. 1875–6

O'Sullivan, Suzanne, *It's All In Your Head: True Stories of Imaginary Illness* (London, 2016)

Porges, Stephen W., *The Polyvagal Theory: Neurophysiological Foundations of Emotion, Attachment, Communication, Self-Regulation* (London, 2011)

Prigogine, Ilya, in collaboration with Isabelle Stengers, *The End of Certainty: Time, Chaos, and the New Laws of Nature* (London, 1997)

Rabin, David, 'Compounding the Ordeal of ALS – Isolation from my Fellow Physicians', *New England Journal of Medicine*, CCCVIII/8 (1982), pp. 506–9

Rabin, Pauline L., and David Rabin, eds, *To Provide Safe Passage: The Humanistic Aspects of Medicine* (New York, 1985)

Rabin, Roni, *Six Parts Love: One Family's Battle with Lou Gehrig's Disease* (New York, 1985)

Rausing, Sigrid, *Mayhem: A Memoir* (London, 2017)

Rawls, Anne Warfield, and Waverly Duck, *Tacit Racism* (London, 2020)

Ricoeur, Paul, *Oneself as Another*, trans. Kathleen Blamey (London, 1992)

Robillard, Albert B., *Meaning of a Disability: The Lived Experience of Paralysis* (Philadelphia, PA, 1999)

Rose, Gillian, *Love's Work* (London, 1994)
—, *Paradiso* (London, 1999)
Rose, Nikolas, and Des Fitzgerald, *The Urban Brain: Mental Health in the Vital City* (Princeton, NJ, 2022)
Schore, Alan N., 'The Interpersonal Neurobiology of Intersubjectivity', *Frontiers in Psychology*, XII (2021), https://doi.org/10.3389/fpsyg.2021.648616
Segal, Julia, *The Trouble with Illness: How Illness and Disability Affect Relationships* (London, 2017)
Sen, Amartya, *Inequality Reexamined* (Oxford, 1992)
Shanahan, Fergus, *The Language of Illness* (Dublin, 2020)
Sontag, Susan, *Illness as Metaphor and AIDS and Its Metaphors* (Harmondsworth, 2000)
Stern, Daniel N., *Forms of Vitality: Exploring Dynamic Experience in Psychology, the Arts, Psychotherapy, and Development* (Oxford, 2010)
—, *The Interpersonal World of the Infant: A View from Psychoanalysis and Developmental Psychology* (New York, 1985, repr. London, 1998)
Szasz, Thomas S., 'The Communication of Distress Between Child and Parent', *Medical Psychology*, XXXII/3 (1959), pp. 161–70
Tolstoy, Leo, *The Death of Ivan Ilyich*, trans. Hugh Aplin (London, 2013)
Tooby, John, and Leda Cosmides, 'Friendship and the Banker's Paradox: Other Pathways to the Evolution of Adaptations for Altruism', *Proceedings of the British Academy*, LXXXVIII (1996), pp. 119–43
Trevarthen, Colwyn, 'Embodied Human Intersubjectivity: Imaginative Agency, to Share Meaning', *Cognitive Semiotics*, IV/1 (2013), pp. 6–56
—, 'Making Sense of Infants Making Sense', *Intellectica*, XXXIV/1 (2002), pp. 161–88
—, '"Stepping Away from the Mirror: Pride and Shame in Adventures of Companionship": Reflections on the Nature and Emotional Needs of Infant Intersubjectivity', in *Attachment and Bonding: A New Synthesis*, ed. C. Sue Carter et al. (London, 2006), pp. 55–84
Tronick, Edward Z., *The Neurobehavioral and Social-Emotional Development of Infants and Children* (New York, 2007)
Van der Kolk, Bessel, *The Body Keeps the Score: Brain, Mind and Body in the Healing of Trauma* (London, 2014)
Wendell, Sarah, 'Unhealthy Disabled: Treating Chronic Illnesses as Disability', *Hypatia*, XVI/4 (2001), pp. 17–33
Whitehead, Anne, and Angela Woods, eds, *The Edinburgh Companion to the Critical Medical Humanities* (Edinburgh, 2016)
Wild, Christopher Paul, 'Complementing the Genome with an "Exposome": The Outstanding Challenge of Environmental Exposure Measurement in Molecular Epidemiology', *Cancer Epidemiology, Biomarkers and Prevention*, XIV/8 (2005), pp. 1847–50
Wittgenstein, Ludwig, *On Certainty*, trans. Denis Paul and G.E.M. Anscombe, ed. G.E.M. Anscombe and G. H. von Wright (Oxford, 1975)

——, *Philosophical Investigations*, trans. G.E.M. Anscombe, ed. G.E.M. Anscombe and R. Rhees (Oxford, 1953)

Young, Iris Marion, *On Female Body Experience: 'Throwing Like a Girl' and Other Essays* (Oxford, 2005)

Youngjin Kang, 'Why Are Dying Individuals Stigmatized and Socially Avoided? Psychological Explanations', *Journal of Social Work in End-of-Life and Palliative Care*, xvii/4 (2021), pp. 317–48

Zola, Irving Kenneth, *Missing Pieces: A Chronicle of Living with a Disability* (Philadelphia, PA, 1982)

——, 'Pathways to the Doctor: From Person to Patient', *Social Science and Medicine*, vii/9 (1973), pp. 677–89

ACKNOWLEDGEMENTS

This book originated as a series of conversations between the two authors about the isolation of the ill which rapidly branched out into related areas. We are heavily indebted to our colleagues at the Centre for the Humanities and Health at King's College London for their searching comments on the project, especially to Brian Hurwitz, its director until 2020, Patrick ffrench, Tania Gergel, Dan Hall-Flavin, Mohammed Aboulleil Rashed, David Stone and Martina Zimmermann.

NV would like to thank colleagues in the English department at King's who read or discussed parts of the book, especially Lisa Appignanesi, Clare Brant, Jon Day, Lizzie Eger, Lara Feigel, Alan Marshall, Ruvani Ranasinha and Max Saunders. NV would like to thank the Humanities Institute at University College Dublin and the Institut la Personne en Medicine at the Université de Paris-Cité for visiting professorships which enabled him to try out the ideas contained in this book in workshops, seminars and lectures before demanding audiences. Particular thanks go to Liz Barrett, Clare Hayes-Brady and Danielle Petherbridge in Dublin and to Isabelle Aujoulat, Céline Lefève, Elise Ricadat, Bernard Pachoud, Karl-Léo Schwering, Sophie Vasset, François Villa and Mi-Kyung Yi in Paris.

NV also thanks Desmond Christy, Helena Cronin, Brian Jacobs, Martina King, John Launer, Christina Lee, Andrew Lees, Allyson Pollock, Columba Quigley, Jamie Rakoczi, Sarah Richmond, Fergus Shanahan, Kate Shorvon, Denis Staunton, Sridhar Venkapaturam and Jamie Whitehead for discussions that sharpened many of the arguments in these pages. Special thanks are reserved for Martin Moloney, this book's severest and best critic, for inspirational discussions at every stage of its development, and for incisive comments on the strengths and weaknesses of our approach. NV also thanks Sarah Nettleton, without whose inspirational support the book might never have been finished.

We acknowledge the indispensable love and support of our families. NV would like to thank his sons Noah Vickers and Sam Vickers, and sister Frances Vickers. NV is especially grateful to Sarah Richmond who was with this book from its beginning and to whom he owes more than he can say.

Finally, this book is dedicated to the memory of Aubrey Sheiham (1936–2015), a giant among health researchers and a great friend and mentor to NV. The book is, among other things, a testament to the vitality of Aubrey's influence – intellectual and moral – which lives on in so many people around the world.

INDEX

4E cognition 22, 198–9, 214

abandonment 126–7, 163–4
  see also pariah syndrome
ace *see* adverse childhood experience
acquaintances 7, 8, 54–5
addiction *see* drug addiction
adoption 174–5
Adorno, Theodor 155
adult communications 89–93
adverse childhood experience (ACE)
  79, 168, 186–8, 190, 211
affect attunement 82
affordances 166, 180, 214
agency 96, 148, 190–99
  see also embodied agency
AIDS 10, 13, 69, 217
Alcott, Alice 42–3, 48
Alexander, Franz 170–71
allopathos 140–41, 142, 144–5
Alon, Uri 177
ALS *see* motor neurone disease (ALS)
Alzheimer's disease 52–3, 61
ancient Greece 152–3
  see also Aristotle
Anda, Robert F. 79, 186, 187, 190
animal genomics 188–9, 192
annihilation 112
Ariès, Philippe 128
Aristotle, *Nicomachean Ethics* 26, 63–4,
  65
attachment theory 171–2

Banker's Paradox 158–9
Bartlett, Frederic 48
  Remembering 38–9
Bauby, Jean-Dominique, *The Diving Bell
  and the Butterfly* 11
Bauman, Zygmunt 46–7, 62, 161
Bayley, John 59, 60, 61

Iris: A Memoir of Iris Murdoch 11, 51–3
Beck, Ulrich, *Risk Society: Towards a
  New Modernity* 148, 149, 150, 151
Beck-Gernsheim, Elisabeth 151
Beebe, Beatrice 29
Benedek, Therese 171
bereavement 25–6, 192
Bernstein, Jay 85–6
Bertalanffy, Ludwig von 176, 197
biomedicine 20, 31, 107, 169, 173–4,
  192–3, 202–3
biopsychosocial model 20–21, 31–2,
  165–8
  sources 168–80
blindness 43–4, 95
Bloch, Ernst 84
blood pressure 133, 171, 185
bodily strangeness 136–45
body, the 30–31, 152–3, 160, 170, 171,
  211
Bollas, Christopher 60
Bolton, Derek 165
Boston Change Process Study Group 30,
  141–3
Boswell, James 129
Bourdieu, Pierre 145, 148–9
Boyer, Anne 7, 37, 45
breast cancer 9, 37, 51, 97, 217
Brin, Sergei 155
Brodkey, Harold 69
Brody, Howard 214–15
Bruner, Jerome 193, 194–5, 196
buddies 10, 217
buffering 166, 183, 194–5
Butler, Sandra, *Cancer in Two Voices* 51,
  217
bystanding 15

Cacioppo, John T. 191
Callard, Felicity 202–3

cancer 7–8, 9, 11, 45–6, 50, 70
see also breast cancer
Canguilhem, Georges 15, 46, 47, 48, 49
Cannon, Walter B. 169–70, 171
cardiovascular disease 42, 181–3, 185, 187
care 15, 18, 28–9, 72–81, 163, 201–2
buffering 166–7
counterculture 217–18
equality 104–5
infants 21–2, 23, 81–9
logic of 117–19
psychosomatic feelings 64–5
volunteers 10
see also mothers
Carel, Havi 95–6
Caspi, Avshalom 189
Cassell, Eric 15, 110, 115–16
catastrophe 26, 57–8, 61, 62, 71
Catholicism 51, 128–9, 130
cells 176, 177–8, 179–80
charity 216–17
Charon, Rita 101–2, 214
children *see* infants
China 215–16
cholesterol 181, 185
Christakis, Nicholas 112–13
chronic physical illness 13–14, 42–3
see also pain
Clare, Eli 44–5
class 181–3
clinicians *see* doctors
Cole, Stephen W. 135, 191
colleagues 9, 122–3, 124–5
communications 89–93, 131–3
compassion 77, 78–9, 111–12, 113, 115–16,
134–5, 143–4
concentration camps 39–40
consciousness 47, 56, 78, 87–8, 195–7
consultation 35–7, 107–10, 163
Conway, Kathlyn 65, 97, 98–9, 143
cooperation 72–3
copying movement 81–3
coregulation 84
Cosmides, Leda 157–9
counterculture 217–18
creativity 68–9
culture 22, 117, 155, 160, 193–4, 215–16

Darley, John M., *The Unresponsive
Bystander: Why Doesn't He Help?* 15
Darwin, Charles, *The Descent of Man* 135
Davis, J. Timothy 197

death 14, 15–16, 30–31, 128–30, 204
dementia 9, 27, 103–4
see also Alzheimer's disease
denial 62, 153–5
see also bereavement; terminal illness
dependence 26, 56, 61, 63, 71, 80, 81
depression-withdrawal reaction 171–3
Dewey, John 201–2
diabetes 42–3, 173, 175, 181
diagnosis 7, 27–8, 37, 96–7, 204–5
doctors 97–8, 107–10
Diamond, John 11
disability 14, 44–5, 49, 94–6, 137
Zola 40–42, 47–8, 100–101, 102
discrimination 13, 44–5
Diving Bell and the Butterfly, The
(film) 11
divorce rates 151
doctors 97–100, 104–5, 167–8
consultation 35–7
pariah syndrome 123–4
patient care 105–10
prognosis 112–16
domestic abuse 67–8
Down's Syndrome 26
drug addiction 53, 61–2
Du Bois, W.E.B. 207
Duck, Waverly 206, 207
Dunbar, Helen Flanders 171
Dunedin Multidisciplinary Health and
Development Study 188, 189
Durkheim, Émile 160–61
*Les formes élémentaires de la vie
religieuse* 91–2
dyadic states 83, 87–9
dying *see* death

E. coli 177–8, 179–80
ecological niches 159–60, 214
Ehrenreich, Barbara 11
Elias, Norbert 204
The Society of Individuals 146–7, 150
embodied agency 166–8, 190–99, 213,
214
embodiment 136–8, 164, 166–7
emergent illness 51–5, 162–3
empathic witness 94, 101–2
employment 48–9, 148, 181–3
see also unemployment
Engel, George 20, 31, 165–6, 167–8, 197
biomedicine 169, 173–4, 175–6
depression-withdrawal 171–3

Index

epidemiology 21, 164–5, 168
see also Whitehall Study
epigenetics 19, 21, 164–5, 168
equality 104–5, 205–6
see also inequality
evolution 135, 204
evolutionary psychology 14, 157–61
eye contact 82, 83

faces 132–3
family members 8, 27, 61–2, 147, 149
see also mothers
Fanon, Frantz 30, 137
Fein, Helen 30, 149
Felitti, Vincent J. 79, 186, 187, 190
feminism 73–5, 76, 137–8
fight–flight response 25, 133, 170
Fisher, Berenice 73–5, 76
Fitzgerald, Des 202–3, 214
Foucault, Michel 46, 49, 155
The Birth of the Clinic 47
Discipline and Punish 48
Fox, John 191
Frank, Arthur W. 9, 10, 49, 50
At the Will of the Body 70
The Wounded Storyteller 18, 215
Freud, Sigmund 57, 58, 172
'Thoughts for the Times on War and Death' 154–5
friendships 7, 8, 9, 27–8, 63–4
Fulton, Robert 153

Garfinkel, Harold 90, 205–6
Garland-Thomson, Rosemarie 42, 48
Gawande, Atul, *Being Mortal* 113–14
genetics 178, 179
see also epigenetics
gesture 131–2
Gibson, James 166, 180
Gilligan, Carol 73
In a Different Voice 74
Girl, Interrupted (film) 11
glucocorticoids 185
Goffman, Erving 23–4, 29, 50
interaction order 80, 90–91, 92–3, 209
Stigma: Notes on the Management of Spoiled Identity 13, 14
Goode, David 53, 60
Gross, Kate 11
groups 34, 35, 37, 38–9, 50–51, 163–4
biological strength 128–36

habitus 145, 147
Hacking, Ian 46, 47, 48, 49, 50
Hadas, Rachel 8, 9
Harari, Yuval Noah, *Sapiens: A Brief History of Humankind* 155–6
harm principle 116–17
Hawking, Stephen 102–3
health 21, 30–31, 150–52, 200–201
inequalities 190–99, 211
interpersonal engagements 164–5
social determinants 19, 181–4
healthcare services 48, 79, 81, 105–20, 147
see also doctors
Heaney, Seamus, 'Miracle' 9
heart disease *see* cardiovascular disease
Hegel, Georg Wilhelm Friedrich 155
Held, Virginia 73
Heliobacter pylori 169
Henrich, Joseph 11–12
high-engagement interaction 24–5, 63
hijackings 40
Hilbert, Richard 69
HIV 13, 217
Hochschild, Arlie Russell 76
The Managed Heart 93–4
Hodges, Brian 66
holding environment 23, 24, 25, 26–7, 28, 51–71, 210–11
care 77, 80
compassion 111–12
mirroring 78, 101, 103
homeostasis 169–70
HPA (hypothalamus-pituitary-adrenaline) axis 185
Hull, John M. 43–4, 95
Hume, David 129, 130
Husserl, Edmund 16–17, 78, 82
hysteria 48

Illich, Ivan, *Medical Nemesis* 204–5
illness 7–9, 11–13, 15, 18–19, 20–21, 34–5, 200–201
death reminder 204
emergent 51–5, 162–3
holding 60–61
isolation 217, 218
normalization 47–8
unmourned losses 67
see also terminal illness; trouble
immortality 155–6
implicit relational knowing 141–3, 144–5, 164

inequality 19, 190–99, 204–5, 211, 218
infants 19, 26, 130–31, 141–2
  adult communications roots 89–93
  care 28–9, 77, 78, 81–9, 167
  culture 193–4
  healthcare 79
  holding 55–8, 59, 61, 66, 68
  neurochemistry 171–2
  research 21–2, 23, 24, 25, 26–7,
    209–10, 214
  systems theory 176–7
  see also adverse childhood experiences
    (ACE)
interaction orders 23–5, 90–93, 205–9
Iris (film) 11
irreplaceability 158–9
isolation 7, 13, 14, 32, 217, 218
  disability 94–6
  evolutionary psychology 157–9,
    160–61
  see also pariah syndrome

Jain, S. Lochlann 7–8

Kaiser Permanente 79, 186
Kanter, Joel 55
Kaysen, Susanna, Girl, Interrupted 11
'keeping people in' 43–4
Kegan, Robert 58–9
Kety, Seymour 174–5
Kleinman, Arthur 72–3, 75, 76, 215–16
  The Illness Narratives 42–3
Kleinman, Joan 215–16
Krieger, Nancy 31
Kübler-Ross, Elisabeth 113, 115
  On Death and Dying: What the Dying
    Have to Teach Doctors, Nurses, Clergy,
    and Their Own Families 15–16
Kugiumutzakis, Giannis 81
Kurzban, Robert 157
Kurzweil, Ray 167

Lamont, Elizabeth 112–13
Laszlo, Ervin 214–15
Latané, Bibb, The Unresponsive Bystander:
    Why Doesn't He Help? 15
Latour, Bruno 117
Leary, Mark R. 157
Lees, Andrew 107–9, 115
letting go 58–9
Levinas, Emmanuel 26, 75–6
  Otherwise than Being 141

Lewontin, Richard 159–60
Link, Bruce 43
London Lighthouse 10
loneliness 13, 25, 191
  see also isolation
Lou Gehrig's disease see motor neurone
    disease (ALS)
Lyons-Ruth, Karlen 142–3

McCrum, Robert 11, 208, 216
Macmillan Cancer Support 50, 217
McRuer, Robert 42
Malloch, Stephen 85
Marmot, Michael 166, 181–2, 183, 191
  The Health Gap 216
marriage 191
Marshall, Barry 169
mass individualization 147
material semiotics 203–4
Meares, Russell 78, 82
Mechanic, David 35
medical students 65–6
medicine 46–7, 165, 166, 202–3
  see also biomedicine
memory 38–9
mental illness 13, 144, 187
  see also schizophrenia
Merleau-Ponty, Maurice 17, 82, 96,
    141
Meyers, Todd 211–13
Mialet, Hélène 103
microsociology 90, 205, 209, 210
minorities 12
mirroring 77–8, 80–81, 89–90, 93–105,
    132
  consultations 108–9
  infants 81–2, 85–7
  reward 92
modernity 30–31, 127–8, 146–57, 160
Mol, Annemarie 79, 81
  The Body Multiple: Ontology in
    Medical Practice 119–20
  The Logic of Care: Health and the
    Problem of Patient Choice 117–19
Monod, Jacques 177, 179
Monopoli, Sara 113–14
mothers 55–7, 66, 84–5, 86–7, 171–2,
    188–9
motor neurone disease (ALS) 9, 12–13,
    53–4, 98–9, 102–3, 121–6, 134
movement 81–5, 90
Murdoch, Iris 11, 51–3, 59, 60, 61

Index

Murphy, Robert F., *The Body Silent* 42, 96–7
musicality 84–5

narrative capacity 194–5
nervous system 25, 133, 143–4
neurology 107–9
neuroscience *see* social neuroscience
neurotransmitters 178–9
Noddings, Nel 73, 74
normalization 34–5, 38–51
    holding 51–71

obligation 30, 149–50
O'Mahoney, Seamus, *The Way We Die Now* 114
omnipotence 15, 16, 17, 71, 211
O'Neill, Desmond 103–4, 105
open systems 176–7, 195
organizing associations 148–9
O'Sullivan, Suzanne 115
otherness 140–41, 142

pain 42, 69
pariah syndrome 12–13, 29–30, 121–6, 134, 143
Parsons, Talcott 51
pathos 138–9, 140–41
peptic ulcers 169
personality types 168–9, 171
Phelan, Jo 43
phenomenology 30, 102
physicians *see* doctors
physiological communication 132–3
physiological embedding adversity 181–9
Picardie, Ruth 11
play 68–9, 80, 86–7, 163
politics 76, 167
Polyvagal Theory 143–5, 164
poor, the 75, 183–4
Porges, Stephen W. 30, 132–3, 143–5, 164
Potter, Dennis 69–70
premature widow syndrome 8, 62
presence 75–6
Price, A. W. 63–4
Prigogine, Ilya 25, 88, 177, 179–80
psychoanalysis 170–71, 175, 197
psychosocial causation 168–9, 181–9, 192–3
psychosomatic feelings 64–6, 71, 112, 211

Rabin, David 12–13, 112, 121–6, 134, 143, 206
    'Isolation from My Fellow Physicians' 99–100
race 137, 207, 212
Rausing, Sigrid 53, 59, 60, 61–2
Rawls, Anne Warfield 206, 207
Redelmeier, Donald 191
Reichsman, Franz 171, 172
relationships 7–10, 23–4, 142–3, 202
    see also friendships
religion 12, 91–2, 134, 151
    see also Catholicism
resilience 130–31, 163–4
reward 85–6, 92
rhesus monkeys 188–9
rhythm 84, 85, 89, 90, 130, 131–2, 133
Ricoeur, Paul 26, 104, 112
ritual 91–2
Robillard, Albert 9, 53–4, 59, 94–5, 102–3, 151
    healthcare professionals 98, 99, 112
Romanian orphans 25
Romano, John 171
Rose, Geoffrey 216
Rose, Gillian 70
Rose, Nikolas 214
Rosenblum, Barbara 136
    Cancer in Two Voices 51, 217
Rosenthal, David 165–6, 174, 175

Sacks, Harvey, 'On Doing "Being Ordinary"' 39–40
safety 101, 132, 133–4, 135, 144–5, 164, 210
Sander, Louis 141
Sapolsky, Robert M. 179
SARS-COV2 pandemic 147, 156
Saunders, Cicely 116
Scarry, Elaine 69
schizophrenia 165–6, 174–5
Schopenhauer, Arthur 155
Schore, Allan 87
Schwamm, Ellen 69
Segal, Hanna 68
Segal, Julia 68
self-holding 60–61, 70
Selye, Hans 170, 171
Sen, Amartya 192
Sennett, Richard 148
    Flesh and Stone: The Body and the City in Western Civilization 152–3
serotonin 188–9, 192

255

shared body schema 17, 82
shared life 21–3
Sheldon, Alan 214–15
Sherrington, Charles, *The Integrative Action of the Nervous System* 139
silence 42
Singh, Sheldon 191
Smith, Adam 129
social connectedness 191–2
social engagement system (SES) 133, 144
social neuroscience 21, 30, 164–5, 168, 210
Sontag, Susan, *Illness as Metaphor* 9
spirituality 44–5, 69–70
stable mirroring 101–2
state, the 146–7
status 190–91
Stengers, Isabelle 25, 177, 179–80
Stern, Daniel N. 29, 81, 84, 87, 141
stigma 8, 9, 13–14, 35, 43–4, 49–50
  see also pariah syndrome
Still Face experiment 88–9
storytelling 18–19
strangeness 136–45, 164
stress 130–31, 165–6, 169–70, 171, 181
  response 184–6
Suomi, Stephen 188
supported autonomy 168, 190–99
symptoms 25, 28, 34, 35–7, 43, 65
  see also diagnosis
systems theory 19, 176–80, 214–15
Szasz, Thomas 17–18

tame death 128–9, 130, 150–51
Taylor, Graeme 172
terminal illness 15–16, 69–70, 112–16
Terrence Higgins Trust 10
Thornicroft, Graham 144
thriving 59–60
tokens of commonality 98–9
Tolstoy, Leo, *The Death of Ivan Ilyich* 153–4, 156
Tooby, John 157–9
transitional experience 68–70, 71, 211
Trevarthen, Colwyn 24, 29, 78, 80, 81, 85, 93
Tronick, Edward Z. 29, 83, 87–8, 101, 141, 195–7
Tronto, Joan C. 73–5, 76–7
trouble 34–5, 41
Trust Conditions 206, 207–8

Type A personalities 168–9, 171

unconsciousness 33, 202, 204, 211–13
unemployment 26, 191
unmourned losses 67, 71, 211

Van der Kolk, Bessel 211
Veblen, Thorstein 204

Waldenfels, Bernhard 30, 138–9, 140–41, 142
'War of the Ghosts, The' (folk tale) 38–9
Warren, Robin 169
We-I Balance 146–7, 149, 150
wealth 181–3, 190
WEIRD societies 11–12, 13, 15, 35, 167
  abandonment 127
  compassion 135, 136
  evolutionary psychology 160
  illness 156–7
  individualism 148
  socioeconomics 183–4
Weiss, Gayle 30
welfare states 48
Wendell, Sarah 14
Whitehall Study 168, 181–4, 185
Winnicott, Donald 23, 24, 26, 27, 28–9, 101
  annihilation 111–12
  'Cure' 104–5, 115
  mother/child relations 55–8, 59
  play 86–7
  transitional experience 68–9, 71
  unconsciousness 204
withdrawal 7, 171–3
Wittgenstein, Ludwig 200
women 48, 73–5, 148
  see also feminism
World Health Organization (WHO) 183, 184, 186, 192

Young, Iris Marion 30
  'Throwing Like a Girl' 137

Zola, Irving 10, 100–101, 102
  Missing Pieces 40–42, 47–8
  'Pathways to the Doctor: From Person to Patient' 36–7
zombie institutions 149